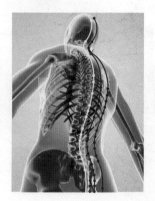

A Manual of State
Standard Acupuncture Points

标准穴位
速学手册

中英文对照真人版

王宏才　王晓珊　王　彤

西安交通大学出版社
XI'AN JIAOTONG UNIVERSITY PRESS

图书在版编目(CIP)数据

标准穴位速学手册/王宏才等编著. —西安:西安
交通大学出版社,2012.6
　ISBN 978 - 7 - 5605 - 3694 - 1

　Ⅰ.①标… Ⅱ.①王… Ⅲ.①穴位疗法-手册
Ⅳ.①R245.9 - 62

　中国版本图书馆 CIP 数据核字(2010)第 164001 号

书　　　名	标准穴位速学手册
编　　　著	王宏才　王晓珊　王　彤
责任编辑	李　晶　张沛烨
出版发行	西安交通大学出版社
	(西安市兴庆南路 10 号　邮政编码 710049)
网　　　址	http://www.xjtupress.com
电　　　话	(029)82668357　82667874(发行中心)
	(029)82668315　82669096(总编办)
传　　　真	(029)82668280
印　　　刷	西安东江印务有限公司
开　　　本	889mm×1194mm　1/48　印张　5
	字数　194 千字
版次印次	2012 年 6 月第 1 版　2012 年 6 月第 1 次印刷
书　　　号	ISBN 978 - 7 - 5605 - 3694 - 1/R・149
定　　　价	25.00 元

读者购书、书店添货、如发现印装质量问题,请与本社发行
中心联系、调换。
订购热线:(029)82665248　(029)82665249
投稿热线:(029)82665546
读者信箱:xjtumpress@163.com

前　言

本书以最新国家标准(GB/T 12346－2008)为依据,收录人体 362 个经穴、46 个经外奇穴及耳穴的标准名称与定位,采用彩色真人照片,将人体体表标志与深层结构准确叠加的图形设计,用不同形式的图形真实、准确、生动、简洁明了的展现腧穴的定位。

书的附录部分为速查部分,分为十四经腧穴名称索引、经外奇穴名称索引和腧穴部位速查。腧穴部位速查即不论是十四经穴,还是经外奇穴,均分部排列,便于读者熟悉腧穴所在部位及相邻腧穴。

全书共配真人彩图百余幅,并配合一些穴位歌诀、常见主治等针灸基础知识,中英文对照,图文互参,方便记忆,易于学习掌握,读者在学习、实践、休闲之余,翻阅本书,定能有所收益。本书适于中医师、中医院校学生、中医爱好者阅读。

《标准穴位速学手册》出版之际,由衷的感谢西安交通大学出版社及编辑等为本书做出的贡献。

Preface

This book is compiled in accordance with the latest national standard (GB/T 12346 - 2008). It includes the standard name and location of 362 meridian points, 46 extraordinary point as well as auricular points. Colour photos of people were adopted together with accurate overlying graphic design of superficial anatomical landmarks and deep structures. Figures of different forms show lively, accurately concisely the location of acupoints.

The appendices of this book are for rapid access, including Index of Acupoints of 14 Meridians, Index of Extra Points, Index of Acupoints in Same Regions. In Index of Acupoints in Same Regions, acupoints of 14 meridians and extraordinary points are listed in one chart if they are located in the same regions so that you can be familiar with not only the location of an acupoint but also its adjacent acupoints in the same region.

This book boasts over 100 colour photos of people and the commonly used indications of acupoints. Annotated in bilinguel Chinese-English, the excellent combination of pictures and language enable you to learn, memorize and master with ease. If you browse this book during your study, practice or spare time, you are bound to benefit from it. If you are a practitioner, a student or an enthusiast of TCM, this book is perfect for you.

On the occasion of the publishing of this book, I would like to express my heartfelt gratefulness to Xi'an Jiaotong University Press and its editors for their contributions to this book.

目 录
CONTENTS

3. 足阳明胃经 Stomach Meridian of Foot Yangming

7. 足太阳膀胱经 Bladder Meridian of Foot Taiyang

8. 足少阴肾经 Kidney Meridian of Foot Shaoyin

11. 足少阳胆经 Gallbladder Meridian of Foot Shaoyang

12. 足厥阴肝经 Liver Meridian of Foot Jueyin

13. 督脉 Governor Vessel

14. 任脉 Conception Vessel

第 3 章　经外奇穴

Chapter III　Extra Points

第 *4* 章　耳穴
Chapter IV　Auricular Points ························ (211)

第 1 章
Chapter I

腧穴的定位
Methods to Locate Acupoints

1. 骨度分寸定位法 Bone Proportional Measurement

骨度分寸定位法是指以体表骨节为主要标志折量全身各部的长度和宽度,定出分寸,用于腧穴定位的方法。即以《灵枢·骨度》规定的人体各部的分寸为基础,并结合历代学者创用的折量分寸(将设定的两骨节点之间的长度折量为一定的等份,每 1 等份为 1 寸,10 等份为 1 尺)作为定穴的依据。

This is a method to locate points on the basis of the distance between the anatomical landmarks. The width or length of various portions of the human body are divided respectively into definite numbers of equal divisions, each division being termed one *cun* . 10 *cun* euqals to 1 *chi*. This method is in accordance with *Chapter of Proportional Measurement in Miraculous Pivot* and the proportions invented by doctors in successive dynasties.

骨度折量寸表　Bone Proportional Measurement

部位 Body part	起止点 Distance	折量寸 Cun	度量法 Method	说明 Explanation
头面部 Head	前发际正中→后发际正中 anterior hairline → posterior hairline	12	直寸 longitudinal measurement	用于确定头部腧穴的纵向距离 longitudinal measurement for the points in the head
	眉间（印堂）→后发际正中→第 7 颈椎棘突下（大椎） Yintang → posterior hair line→Dazhui	18	直寸 longitudinal measurement	用于确定头部及颈后部腧穴的纵向距离 longitudinal measurement for the points in the head and the back of the neck
	两额角发际（头维）之间 between the two corners of anterior hairline	9	横寸 transverse measurement	用于确定头前部腧穴的横向距离 transverse measurement for the points in the forehead
	耳后两乳突（完骨）之间 between the two mastoid processes	9	横寸 transverse measurement	用于确定头后部腧穴的横向距离 transverse measurement for the points in the occiput

部位 Body part	起止点 Distance	折量寸 Cun	度量法 Method	说明 Explanation
胸腹胁部 Chest and Abdomen	胸骨上窝（天突）→胸剑联合中点（歧骨） suprasternal fossa → the middle of sternalcostal angle	9	直寸 longitudinal measurement	用于确定胸部任脉腧穴的纵向距离 longitudinal measurement for the points of Conception Vessel
	胸剑联合中点（歧骨）→脐中 the middle of sternalcostal angle → center of umbilicus	8	直寸 longitudinal measurement	用于确定上腹部腧穴的纵向距离 longitudinal measurement for the points in the upper abdomen
	脐中→耻骨联合上缘（曲骨） center of umbilicus → the upper border of symphysis pubis	5	直寸 longitudinal measurement	用于确定下腹部腧穴的纵向距离 longitudinal measurement for the points in the lower abdomen
	两肩胛骨喙突内侧缘之间 between the medial border of scapula coracoid	12	横寸 transverse measurement	用于确定胸部腧穴的横向距离 transverse measurement for the points in the chest
	两乳头之间 between the two nipples	8	横寸 transverse measurement	用于确定胸腹部腧穴的横向距离 transverse measurement for the points in the chest and abdomen

续表

部位 Body part	起止点 Distance	折量寸 Cun	度量法 Method	说明 Explanation
背腰部 Back	肩胛骨内侧缘→后正中线 the medial border of scapula → the posterior midline	3	横寸 transverse measurement	用于确定背腰部腧穴的横向距离 transverse measurement for the points in the back
上肢部 Upper Limbs	腋前、后纹头→肘横纹（平尺骨鹰嘴） the end of axillary fold → the transverse cubital crease	9	直寸 longitudinal measurement	用于确定上臂部腧穴的纵向距离 longitudinal measurement for the points in the upper arm
	肘横纹（平尺骨鹰嘴）→腕掌（背）侧远端横纹 the transverse cubital crease →the distal transverse wrist crease	12	直寸 longitudinal measurement	用于确定前臂部腧穴的纵向距离 longitudinal measurement for the points in the forearm
下肢部 Lower Limbs	耻骨联合上缘→髌底 the level of upper border of symphysis pubis → the upper border of patella	18	直寸 longitudinal measurement	用于确定大腿部腧穴的纵向距离 longitudinal measurement for the points in the thigh
	髌底→髌尖 the lower border of patella → center of patella	2	直寸 longitudinal measurement	用于确定髌骨周围腧穴的纵向距离 longitudinal measurement for the points around patella
	髌尖（膝中）→内踝尖 apex patella → tip of medial malleolus	15	直寸 longitudinal measurement	用于确定小腿内侧部腧穴的纵向距离 longitudinal measurement for the points in the medial aspect of leg

部位 Body part	起止点 Distance	折量寸 Cun	度量法 Method	说明 Explanation
下肢部 Lower Limbs	胫骨内侧髁下方（阴陵泉）→内踝尖 lower border of medial condyle of tibia → tip of medial malleolus	13	直寸 longitudinal measurement	用于确定小腿内侧部腧穴的纵向距离 longitudinal measurement for the points in the medial aspect of the leg
	股骨大转子→髌横纹（平髌尖） prominence of great trochanter → the center of patella	19	直寸 longitudinal measurement	用于确定大腿部前外侧部腧穴的纵向距离 longitudinal measurement for the points in the anterior or lateral aspect of the thigh
	臀沟→腘横纹 gluteal crease → transverse crease of the popliteal fossa	14	直寸 longitudinal measurement	用于确定大腿后部腧穴的纵向距离 longitudinal measurement for the points in the posterior aspect of the thigh
	腘横纹（平髌尖）→外踝尖 transverse crease of the popliteal fossa → tip of external malleolus	16	直寸 longitudinal measurement	用于确定小腿外侧部腧穴的纵向距离 longitudinal measurement for the points in the lateral aspect of the leg
	内踝尖→足底 tip of medial malleolus → sole of foot	3	直寸 longitudinal measurement	用于确定足内侧部腧穴的纵向距离 longitudinal measurement for the points in the medial aspect of the foot

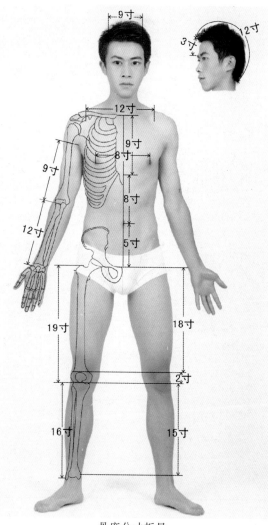

骨度分寸折量

正面,侧面

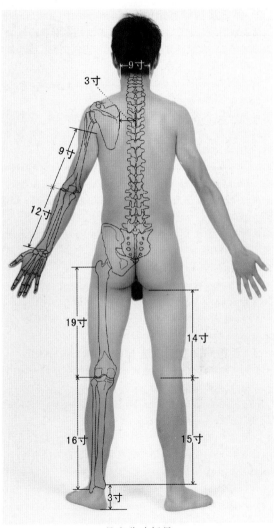

骨度分寸折量
背面

2. 体表解剖标志定位法 Anatomical Landmarks

体表解剖标志定位法是以人体解剖学的各种体表标志为依据来确定腧穴位置的方法,又称自然标志定位法。分为固定的标志和活动的标志两种。

Various anatomical landmarks, fixed and moving on the body surface are taken to help locate acupoints.

➤ 固定的标志:指各部位由骨节、肌肉所形成的突起、凹陷及五官轮廓、发际、指(趾)甲、乳头、肚脐等,是在自然姿势下可见的标志,可以借助这些标志确定腧穴的位置。

Fixed landmarks are those that would not change with body movement, including prominence and depression of bones and muscles, outline of five sense organs, hairlines, nails, nipple, umbilicus, etc.

➤ 活动的标志:指各部的关节、肌肉、肌腱、皮肤随着活动而出现的空隙、凹陷、皱纹、尖端等,是在活动姿势下才会出现的标志,据此亦可确定腧穴的位置。

Moving landmarks are those that will appear only when a body part keeps in a specific position, including cleft, depression, fold, tips, etc. They appear when joints, muscles, tendons, and skin are in a certain position.

3. 手指同身寸定位法 Finger Measurement

手指同身寸定位法是以患者本人手指所规定的分寸以量取腧穴的方法,又称指寸法。

The length and breadth of the patient's finger are used as a criterion for locating acupoints.

➤ 中指同身寸:是以患者的中指中节屈曲时桡侧两端纹头之间作为 1 寸,可用于四肢部阳经的直寸和背部取穴的横寸。

When the middle finger is flexed, the distance between the two ends of the creases of the interphalangeal joints is taken as one cun. This is for longitudinal measurement of the points of yang meridians in the four limbs and transverse measurement of the points in the back.

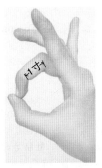

中指同身寸

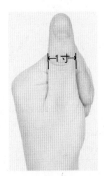

拇指同身寸

> 拇指同身寸:是以患者拇指指间关节的宽度作为 1 寸,亦可用于四肢部的直寸取穴。

The breadth of the interphalangeal joint of thumb is taken as one cun. This is for longitudinal measurement of the points in the four limbs.

> 横指同身寸:又名一夫法,是令患者将食指、中指、无名指和小指并拢,以中指中节横纹处为准,四指横量的宽度作为 3 寸,用于四肢部及腹部的取穴。

The breadth of thefour fingers (index, middle, ring, and little fingers) close together at the level of the skin crease of the proximal interphalangeal joint at the dorsum of the middle finger is taken as 3 cun. This is for points in the four limbs and the abdomen.

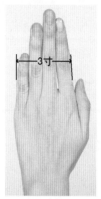

横指同身寸

附:特定穴名称

井穴:Jing-Well point

荥穴:Ying-Spring point

输穴:Shu-Stream point

经穴:Jing-River point

合穴:He-Sea point

原穴:Yuan-Primary point

募穴:Front-Mu point

络穴:Luo-Connecting point

郄穴:Xi-Cleft point

背俞穴:Back-Shu point

下合穴:Lower He-Sea point

八会穴:Eight influential point

八脉交会穴:Eight confluent point

第 2 章
Chapter Ⅱ

十四经腧穴
Acupoints of 14 Meridians

1. 手太阴肺经 Lung Meridian of Hand Taiyin

手太阴肺经分寸歌

乳上三肋间中府，上行一寸云门连。

云在璇玑旁六寸，天府三寸在腋前。

肘上五寸侠白位，尺泽肘横纹中诠。

孔最腕侧上七寸，列缺寸半腕侧边。

经渠腕横纹一寸，太渊掌后横纹联。

鱼际节后白肉际，少商拇甲内侧沿。

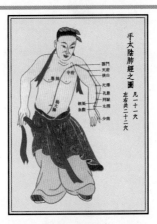

手太阴肺经之图　凡一十一穴　左右共二十二穴

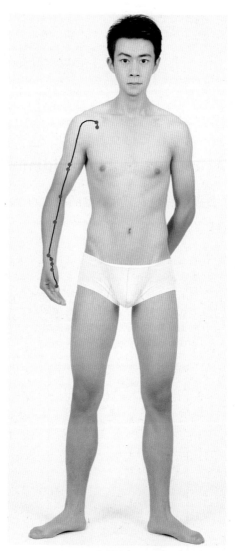

手太阴肺经

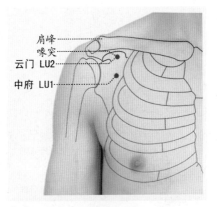

肩峰
喙突
云门 LU2
中府 LU1

LU1 中府 ZhōngFǔ (肺募穴)

位置 胸部,横平第 1 肋间隙,锁骨下窝外侧,前正中线旁开 6 寸。

主治 咳嗽,气喘,胸部胀满,胸痛,肩背痛。

Location：at the level of the first intercostals space, lateral to the infraclavicular fossa, 6 cun lateral to the anterior midline.

Indications：cough, asthma, distending pain in the chest, pain in the shoulder and back.

LU2 云门 YúnMén

位置 胸部,锁骨下窝凹陷处,肩胛骨喙突上方,前正中线旁开 6 寸。

简易取穴 两手叉腰,取正坐坐姿,胸廓上部锁骨外侧端下缘的三角形凹窝正中处即是本穴。

主治 咳嗽,气喘,胸痛,肩背痛。

Location：in the depression of the infraclavicular fossa, at the medial border of scapular coracoid process, 6 cun lateral to the anterior midline. When a person sits bolt upright with arms akimbo, it is in the triangular fossa inferior to the lateral end of the clavicle.

Indications：cough, asthma, pain in the shoulder and back.

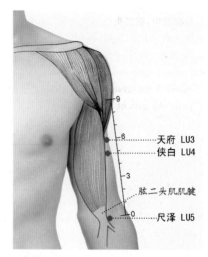

天府 LU3
侠白 LU4
肱二头肌肌腱
尺泽 LU5

LU3 天府 TiānFǔ

位置 臂前区,腋前纹头下 3 寸,肱二头肌桡侧缘处。

简易取穴 取坐位,臂向前平举,俯头鼻尖接触上臂内侧处即是本穴。

主治 气喘,鼻衄,上臂痛。

Location：in the medial aspect of upper arm, 3 cun below the end of the axillary fold, at the radial side of m. biceps brachii. When a person sits, raises the arm horizontally forward, lowers the head, it is where the tip of nose touches the medial aspect of upper arm.

Indications：asthma, epistaxis, pain in the upper arm.

LU4 侠白 XiáBái

位置 臂前区,腋前纹头下 4 寸,肱二头肌桡侧缘。

主治 咳嗽,上臂痛。

Location：in the medial aspect of upper arm, 4 cun below the end of the axillary fold, at the radial side of m. biceps brachii.

Indications：cough, asthma, pain in the upper arm.

LU5 尺泽 ChiZé (合穴)

位置　肘区,肘横纹中,肱二头肌腱桡侧缘凹陷中。

主治　咳嗽,咳血,气喘,咽喉肿痛,小儿惊风,肘臂挛痛。

Location: in the transverse cubital crease, in the depression at the radial side of m. biceps brachii.

Indications: cough, hemoptysis, asthma, sore throat, infantile convulsion, spasmodic pain of the elbow and arm.

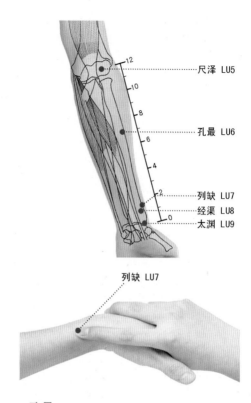

尺泽 LU5

孔最 LU6

列缺 LU7
经渠 LU8
太渊 LU9

列缺 LU7

LU6 孔最 KǒngZuì (郄穴)

位置 前臂前区,腕掌侧远端横纹上 7 寸,尺泽(LU5)与太渊 (LU9)连线上。

主治 咳嗽,气喘,咳血,咽喉肿痛,肘臂挛痛。

Location: in the palmar aspect of the forearm, 7 cun above the distal transverse crease of wrist, in the line connecting ChǐZé (LU5) and TàiYuān (LU9).

Indications: cough, asthma, hemoptysis, sore throat, spasmodic pain of the elbow and arm.

LU7 列缺 LièQuē (络穴、八脉交会穴)

位置 前臂,腕掌侧远端横纹上 1.5 寸,肱桡肌与拇长展肌腱之间,拇长展肌腱沟的凹陷中。

简易取穴 两手虎口交叉,一手食指按在桡骨茎突上,指尖下凹陷中是穴。

主治 头痛,项强,咳嗽,气喘,咽喉肿痛,口眼歪斜。

Location: 1.5 cun proximal to the dorsal transverse crease of wrist, between the tendons of musculus extensor pollicis brachioradials and longus, in the groove of the tendon of musculus extensor pollicis longus. When the index fingers and thumbs of both hands are crossed with the index finger of one hand placed on the styloid process of the radius of the other hand, it is in the depression under the tip of the index finger.

Indications: headache, migraine, neck rigidity, cough, asthma, sore throat, facial paralysis.

LU8 经渠 JīngQú (经穴)

位置 前臂前区,腕掌侧远端横纹上 1 寸,桡骨茎突与桡动脉之间。

简易取穴 脉诊时中指所在的位置即是本穴。

主治 咳嗽,气喘,胸痛,咽喉肿痛,手腕痛。

Location: 1 cun proximal to the distal transverse crease of wrist, between the styloid process of radius and the radial artery. It is just where the middle finger is place in feeling the pulse.

Indications: cough, asthma, sore throat, pain in the wrist.

LU9 太渊 TàiYuān (输穴、原穴、脉会穴)

位置 腕掌横纹桡侧,桡动脉搏动处。

主治 咳嗽,气喘,腕臂痛。

Location: It is in the radial side of the transverse crease of wrist, at where the radial artery beats.

Indications: cough, asthma, pain in the wrist and arm.

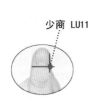

少商 LU11

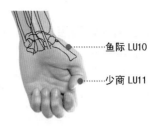

鱼际 LU10

少商 LU11

LU10 鱼际 YúJì（荥穴）

位置　手外侧，第 1 掌骨桡侧中点赤白肉际处。

主治　咳嗽，咯血，咽喉肿痛，失音。

Location：at the midpoint in the radial aspect of the first metacarpal bone, at the junction of red and white skin (i. e. the junction of the dorsum and palm of hand).

Indications：cough, hemoptysis, sore throat, loss of voice, fever, hot sensation in the palm.

LU11 少商 ShàoShāng（井穴）

位置　手指，拇指末节桡侧，指甲根角侧上方 0.1 寸（指寸）。

主治　咽喉肿痛，鼻衄，发热，昏厥，癫狂。

Location：in the radial side of the terminal phalanx of thumb, about 0.1 cun form the corner of nail.

Indications：sore throat, epistaxis, fever, loss of consciousness, mental disorder.

2. 手阳明大肠经 Large Intestine Meridian of Hand Yangming

手阳明大肠经分寸歌

食指甲角取商阳，二间本节前中量。
三间节后依次取，合谷虎口歧骨详。
腕上筋间阳溪位，偏历交差中指行。
温溜腕后去五寸，肘下四寸下廉方。
肘下三寸上廉穴，肘下二寸三里乡。
曲池曲肘纹尺取，肘髎大骨外廉商。
五里距肘上三寸，臂臑肘上七寸望。
肩髃肩端举臂取，巨骨肩尖骨陷藏。
天鼎扶突下一寸，扶突迎后寸半长。
禾髎水沟旁半寸，鼻翼旁边取迎香。

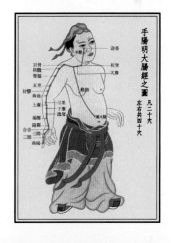

手陽明大腸經之圖

凡二十六 左右共四十六

迎香
扶突
天鼎
巨骨
肩髃
臂臑
五里
曲池
肘髎
上廉
三里 下廉 温溜
偏历
合谷
三间
二间
商阳

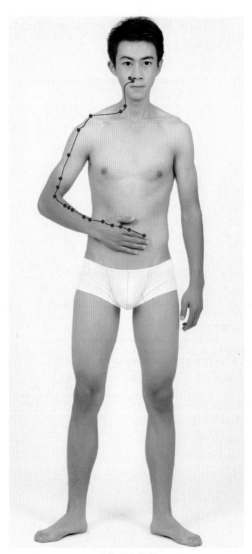

手阳明大肠经

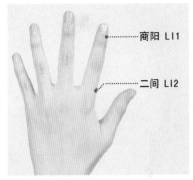

商阳 LI1

二间 LI2

LI1 商阳 ShāngYáng（井穴）

位置　手指,食指末节桡侧,指甲根角侧上方0.1寸(指寸)。

主治　齿痛,咽喉肿痛,热病,昏迷。

Location：in the radial side of the terminal phalanx of index finger, 0.1 cun from the corner of nail.

Indications：toothache, sore throat, febrile disease, loss of consciousness.

LI2 二间 ÈrJiān（荥穴）

位置　手指,第2掌指关节桡侧远端赤白肉际处。

主治　鼻衄,齿痛,热病。

Location：distal to the radial side of the second metacarpophalangeal joint, at the junction of the red and white skin.

Indications：dizziness, epistaxis, toothache, sore throat, febrile disease.

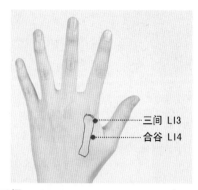

三间 LI3
合谷 LI4

LI3 三间 SānJiān (输穴)

位置　手背,第 2 掌指关节桡侧近端凹陷中。

主治　齿痛,咽喉肿痛。

Location：in the dorsum of hand, in the depression proximal to the radial side of the second metacarpophalangeal joint.

Indications：toothache, ophthalmalgia, sore throat, redness and swelling of fingers and dorsum of hand.

LI4 合谷 HéGǔ (原穴)

位置　手背,第 2 掌骨桡侧的中点处。

主治　头痛,颈项痛,目赤肿痛,鼻衄,鼻塞,齿痛,耳聋,咽喉肿痛,疟腮,口眼歪斜,热病无汗,多汗,闭经,滞产。

Location：in the dorsum of hand, at midpoint in the radial side the second metacarpal bone.

Indications：headache, neck pain, redness, swelling and pain of the eye, epistaxis, nasal obstruction, toothache, deafness, sore throat, parotitis, facial paralysis, febrile diseases with anhidrosis, hidrosis, amenorrhea, prolonged labour.

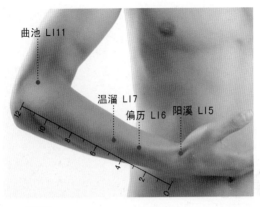

曲池 LI11
温溜 LI7
偏历 LI6
阳溪 LI5

LI5 阳溪 YángXī (经穴)

位置 腕区,腕背侧远端横纹桡侧,当拇短伸肌腱与拇长伸肌腱之间的凹陷处。

主治 头痛,目赤肿痛,手腕痛。

Location: at the radial side in the dorsal distal crease of wrist, in the depression proximal between the tendons of musculus extensor pollicis brevis and longus.

Indications: headache, redness, pain in the wrist.

LI6 偏历 PiānLì (络穴)

位置 前臂,腕背侧远端横纹上 3 寸,阳溪(LI5)与曲池(LI11)连线上。

主治 耳鸣,鼻衄,手臂酸痛。

Location: 3 cun proximal the dorsal distal crease of wrist, in the line connecting YángXī (LI5) and QǔChí (LI11).

Indications: tinnitus, epistaxis.

LI7 温溜 WēnLiū (郄穴)

位置 前臂,腕背侧远端横纹上 5 寸,阳溪(LI5)与曲池(LI11)连线上。

主治 头痛,面肿,咽喉肿痛,肠鸣。

Location: 5 cun proximal the dorsal distal crease of wrist, in the line connecting YángXī (LI5) and QǔChí (LI11).

Indications: headache, facial swelling, sore throat, borborygmus.

曲池 LI11
手三里 LI10
上廉 LI9
下廉 LI8
阳溪 LI5

LI8 下廉 XiàLián

位置 前臂,肘横纹下 4 寸,阳溪(LI5)与曲池(LI11)连线上。

主治 腹痛,肘臂痛,上肢不遂。

Location:4 cun distal to the transverse cubital crease, in the line connecting YángXī (LI5) and QǔChí (LI11).

Indications:abdominal pain, pain in the elbow and arm, motor impairment of the upper limbs.

LI9 上廉 ShàngLián

位置 前臂,肘横纹下 3 寸,阳溪(LI5)与曲池(LI11)连线上。

主治 肘臂疼痛,上肢不遂,手臂麻木,肠鸣、腹痛。

Location:3 cun distal to the transverse cubital crease, in the line connecting YángXī (LI5) and QǔChí (LI11).

Indications:pain in the shoulder and arm, motor impairment of the upper limbs, numbness of arm, borborygmus, abdominal pain.

LI10 手三里 ShǒuSānLi

位置 前臂,肘横纹下 2 寸,阳溪(LI5)与曲池(LI11)连线上。

主治 腹痛,腹泻,齿痛,颊肿,上肢不遂。

Location:2 cun distal to the transverse cubital crease, in the line connecting YángXī (LI5) and QǔChí (LI11).

Indications:abdominal pain, diarrhea, toothache, swelling of the cheek, motor impairment of the upper limbs.

LI11 曲池 QūChí (合穴)

位置 肘区,肘横纹外侧端与肱骨外上髁连线的中点处。

主治 咽喉肿痛,齿痛,目赤痛,瘰疬,风疹,上肢不遂,腹痛,吐泻,热病。

Location: at the lateral end of the transverse cubital crease, midway between the radial side of the transverse cubital crease and the lateral epicondyle of the humerus

Indications: sore throat, toothache, redness and swelling of the eye, scrofula, urticaria, motor impairment of the upper limbs, abdominal pain with vomiting and diarrhea, febrile disease.

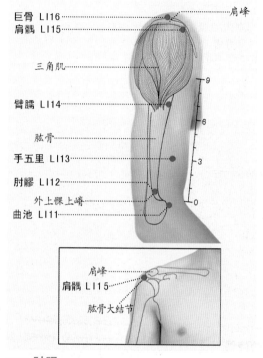

巨骨 LI16
肩髃 LI15
肩峰
三角肌
臂臑 LI14
肱骨
手五里 LI13
肘髎 LI12
外上髁上嵴
曲池 LI11

9
6
3
0

肩峰
肩髃 LI15
肱骨大结节

LI12 肘髎 ZhǒuLiáo

位置　肘区,肱骨外上髁上缘,髁上嵴的前缘。

主治　肘臂疼痛、麻木、挛急。

Location：proximal to the lateral epicondyle of humerus, at the anterior border of supracondylar ridge.

Indications：pain, spasm or numbness of the elbow and arm.

LI13 手五里 ShǒuWǔLǐ

位置　臂部,肘横纹上 3 寸,曲池(LI11)与肩髃(LI15)连线上。

主治　肘臂挛痛,瘰疬。

Location：3 cun proximal to the transverse cubital crease, in the line connecting QǔChí (LI11) and JiānYú (LI15).

Indications：pain and spasm of the elbow and arm，scrofula.

LI14 臂臑 BìNào

位置 臂部,曲池(LI11)上 7 寸,三角肌前缘处。

主治 肩臂痛,颈项拘急,瘰疬。

Location：7 cun proximal to QǔChí（LI11），in the anterior border of m. deltoideus.

Indications：pain of the shoulder and arm，spasm of neck，scrofula.

LI15 肩髃 JiānYú

位置 三角肌区,肩峰外侧缘前端与肱骨大结节两骨间凹陷中。

主治 肩臂疼痛,上肢不遂,隐疹。

Location：in the depression between the anterior lateral aspect of acromion and the greater tubercle of humerus.

Indications：pain of shoulder and arm，motor impairment of the upper limbs，urticaria.

LI16 巨骨 JùGǔ

位置 肩胛区,锁骨肩峰端与肩胛冈之间凹陷中。

主治 肩臂疼痛,抬举不利,肩背痛,瘰疬。

Location：in the upper aspect of shoulder，in the depression between the acromial extremity of clavicle and the scapular spine.

Indications：pain and motor impairment of the shoulder and arm，back pain，scrofula.

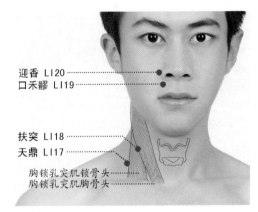

迎香 LI20
口禾髎 LI19

扶突 LI18
天鼎 LI17

胸锁乳突肌锁骨头
胸锁乳突肌胸骨头

LI

LI17 天鼎 TiānDǐng

位置　颈部,横平环状软骨,胸锁乳突肌后缘。

主治　暴喑,咽喉肿痛,瘰疬,瘿气。

Location：in the lateral side of neck, at the level of the annular cartilage, in the posterior border of m. sternocleidomastoideus

Indications：loss of voice, sore throat, scrofula, goiter.

LI18 扶突 FúTū

位置　胸锁乳突肌区,横平喉结,胸锁乳突肌前、后缘中间。

主治　咳嗽,气喘,咽喉肿痛,暴喑,瘰疬,瘿气。

Location：at the level of the tip of prominentia laryngea, between the sternal head and clavicular head of m. sternocleidomastoideus.

Indications：cough, asthma, sore throat, loss of voice, scrofula, goiter.

LI19 口禾髎 KǒuHéLiáo

位置　面部,横平人中沟上 1/3 与下 2/3 交点,鼻孔外缘直下。

主治　鼻塞,鼻衄,口歪。

Location：at the level of the junction of upper one—third and lower two—thirds of philtrum, directly below the lateral margin of nostril

Indications：nasal obstruction, epistaxis, deviation of mouth.

LI20 迎香 YíngXiāng

位置　面部,鼻翼外缘中点旁,鼻唇沟中。

主治　鼻塞,鼻衄,鼻渊,口歪。

Location：in the nasolabial groove, at the level of the midpoint of the lateral border of ala nasi.

Indications：nasal obstruction, epistaxis, rhinorrhea, deviation of mouth, facial swelling.

3. 足阳明胃经 Stomach Meridian of Foot Yangming

足阳明胃经分寸歌

足之经兮阳明胃，承泣目下七分详。

四白目下一寸取，巨髎八分鼻孔旁。

地仓挟吻四分近，大迎颔前寸三乡。

颊车耳下曲颊陷，下关耳前动脉行。

头维神庭旁四五，人迎喉旁寸五量。

水突筋前迎下在，气舍突下穴相当。

缺盆舍外横骨内，相去中行四寸量。

气户璇玑旁四寸，至乳六寸四分方。

库房屋翳膺窗近，乳中下在乳头心。

次有乳根出乳下，名一寸六不相侵。

却去中行须四寸，胸膺穴位要细斟。

不容巨阙旁二寸，去近幽门寸五存。

其下承满与梁门，关门太乙滑肉门。

上下一寸无多少，共去中行二寸寻。

天枢脐旁二寸间，枢下三寸水道传。

水下一寸归来好，距离中行二寸边。

气冲鼠蹊上一寸，又距中行二寸间。

髀关膝上有尺二，伏兔膝上六寸焉。

阴市膝上方三寸，梁丘膝上二寸施。

膝膑陷中犊鼻穴，膝下三寸三里施。

上廉在膝下六寸，膝下八寸条口寻。

膝下九寸下廉是，踝上八寸丰隆安。

解溪跗上系鞋处，踝骨横纹中央观。

冲阳跗上五寸唤，陷谷庭后二寸间。

内庭次趾外间陷，厉兑足次趾外端。

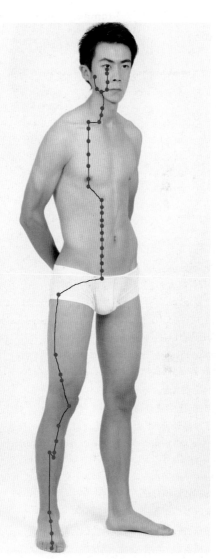

足阳明胃经

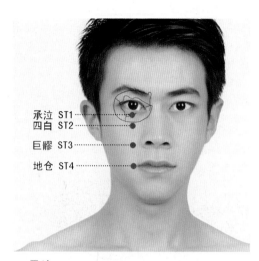

承泣　ST1
四白　ST2
巨髎　ST3
地仓　ST4

ST1 承泣 ChéngQì

位置　面部,眼球与眶下缘之间,瞳孔直下。

主治　目赤肿痛,流泪,夜盲,口眼歪斜。

Location: between the eyeball and the midpoint of infraorbital ridge, directly below the pupil.

Indications: redness, swelling and pain of the eye, lacrimation induced by wind, night blindness, facial paralysis.

ST2 四白 SìBái

位置　面部,眶下孔处,瞳孔直下。

主治　目赤痛痒,口眼歪斜,面痛。

Location: in the depression at the infraorbital foramen, directly below the pupil.

Indications: redness, itching and pain of the eye, facial paralysis, trigeminal neuralgia.

ST3 巨髎 JùLiáo

位置　面部,横平鼻翼下缘处,瞳孔直下。

主治　口眼歪斜,鼻衄,齿痛,唇颊肿。

Location: at the level of the lower border of ala nasi, directly below the pupil.

Indications：facial paralysis，epistaxis，toothache，swelling of lips and cheek.

ST4 地仓 DìCāng

位置 面部，口角旁开 0.4 寸(指寸)，瞳孔直下。

主治 口角歪斜，流涎。

Location：0.4 cun (finger measurement) lateral to the corner of mouth，directly below the pupil.

Indications：facial paralysis，hypersalivation.

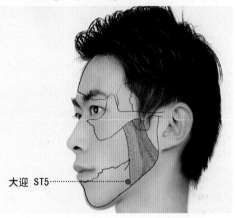

大迎 ST5

ST5 大迎 DàYíng

位置 面部，下颌角前方，咬肌附着部的前缘凹陷中，面动脉搏动处。

主治 口眼歪斜，颊肿，面痛，齿痛。

Location：anterior to the angle of mandible，in the depression at the anterior border of attachment of m. masseter，at where the facial artery beats.

Indications：facial paralysis，swelling of cheek，trigeminal neuralgia，toothache.

头维 ST8

下关 ST7

颊车 ST6

ST6 颊车 JiáChē

位置 面部,下颌角前上方一横指(中指)。

注:沿下颌角角平分线上一横指,闭口咬紧牙时咬肌隆起处,放松时按之有凹陷处。

主治 口眼歪斜,齿痛,颊肿,面肿,疟腮,牙关紧闭。

Location:one finger-breadth(middle finger)superior to the angle of mandible where m. masseter attaches at the prominence of the muscle when the teeth are clenched.

Indications:facial paralysis,toothache,swelling of the cheek or face,parotitis,trismus.

ST7 下关 XiàGuān

位置 面部,颧弓下缘中央与下颌切迹之间凹陷中。

主治 耳聋,耳鸣,齿痛,口眼歪斜,面痛,牙关开合不利。

Location:in the depression between the midpoint of the lower border of the zygomatic arch and mandibular incisure.

Indications:deafness,tinnitus,toothache,facial paralysis,trigeminal neuralgia,motor impairment of the jaw.

ST8 头维 TóuWéi

位置 头部,额角发际直上 0.5 寸,头正中线旁开 4.5 寸。

主治 头痛,目眩,目痛。

Location:0.5 cun within the anterior hairline at the corner of the forehead,4.5 cun lateral to the anterior midline.

Indications:headache,blurred vision,ophthalmalgia.

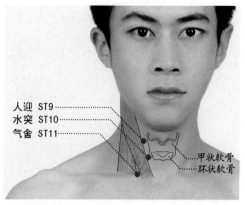

人迎 ST9
水突 ST10
气舍 ST11

甲状软骨
环状软骨

ST9 人迎 RénYíng

位置 颈部,横平结喉,胸锁乳突肌前缘,颈总动脉搏动处。

主治 咽喉肿痛,气喘,瘿气,眩晕。

Location:at the level of the tip of prominentia laryngea, in the anterior border of m. sternocleidomastoideus, at where the common carotid artery beats.

Indications:sore throat, asthmatic breathing, goiter, dizziness, flushing of face.

ST10 水突 ShuǐTū

位置 颈部,横平环状软骨,胸锁乳突肌前缘。

主治 咽喉肿痛,气喘,咳嗽。

Location:at the level of the annular cartilage, in the anterior border of m. sternocleidomastoideus.

Indications:sore throat, asthmatic breathing, cough.

ST11 气舍 QìShě

位置 胸锁乳突肌区,锁骨上小窝,锁骨胸骨端上缘,胸锁乳突肌胸骨头与锁骨头中间的凹陷中。

主治 咽喉肿痛,颈部强痛,气喘,呃逆,瘿瘤。

Location:at the superior border of the sternal extremity of the clavicle, in the depression between the sternal head and clavicular head of m. sternocleidomastoideus.

Indications:sore throat, stiffness and pain of the neck, asthmatic breathing, hiccup, goiter.

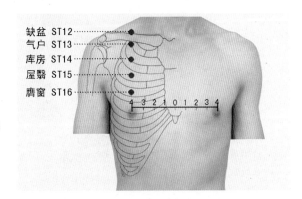

缺盆 ST12
气户 ST13
库房 ST14
屋翳 ST15
膺窗 ST16

ST12 缺盆 QuēPén

位置 颈外侧区,锁骨上大窝,锁骨上缘凹陷中,前正中线旁开4寸。

主治 咳嗽,气喘,咽喉肿痛,缺盆中痛。

Location:at the midpoint of the supraclavicular fossa, 4 cun lateral to the anterior midline.

Indications:cough, asthmatic breathing, sore throat, pain in the supraclavicular fossa.

ST13 气户 QìHù

位置 胸部,锁骨下缘,前正中线旁开4寸。

主治 胸部胀满,气喘,咳嗽,呃逆,胸胁痛。

Location:in the chest, at the lower border of the middle of clavicle, 4 cun lateral to the anterior midline.

Indications:fullness in the chest, asthmatic breathing, cough, hiccup, pain in the hypochondrium.

ST14 库房 KùFáng

位置 胸部,第1肋间隙,前正中线旁开4寸。

主治 胸胁胀痛,咳嗽。

Location:in the first intercostal space, 4 cun lateral to the anterior midline.

Indications:distending pain in the chest and hypochondrium, cough.

ST15 屋翳 WūYì

位置 胸部,第 2 肋间隙,前正中线旁开 4 寸。

主治 胸胁胀痛,咳嗽,气喘,乳痈。

Location: in the second intercostal space, 4 cun lateral to the anterior midline.

Indications: distending pain in the chest and hypochondrium, cough, asthmatic breathing, mastitis.

ST16 膺窗 YīngChuāng

位置 胸部,第 3 肋间隙,前正中线旁开 4 寸。

主治 胸胁胀痛,咳嗽,气喘,乳痈。

Location: in the third intercostal space, 4 cun lateral to the anterior midline.

Indications: distending pain in the chest and hypochondrium, cough, asthmatic breathing, mastitis.

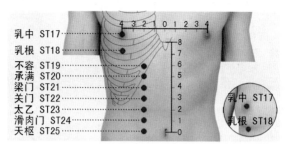

乳中	ST17
乳根	ST18
不容	ST19
承满	ST20
梁门	ST21
关门	ST22
太乙	ST23
滑肉门	ST24
天枢	ST25

乳中 ST17
乳根 ST18

ST17 乳中 RǔZhōng

位置 胸部,乳头中央。

注:本穴不针不灸,只作定位标志。

Location:in the center of the nipple.

Note:Prohibit puncture and moxa,just as marker of location.

ST18 乳根 RǔGēn

位置 胸部,第5肋间隙,前正中线旁开4寸。

主治 胸痛,咳嗽,气喘,乳痈,乳汁少。

Location:in the fifth intercostal space,4 cun lateral to the anterior midline.

Indications:chest pain,cough,asthmatic breathing,mastitis,insufficient lactation.

ST19 不容 BùRóng

位置 上腹部,脐中上6寸,前正中线旁开2寸。

主治 腹胀,呕吐,胃痛,食欲不振。

Location:in the upper abdomen,6 cun above the umbilicus,2 cun lateral to the anterior midline.

Indications:abdominal distension,vomiting,gastric pain,poor appetite.

ST20 承满 ChéngMǎn

位置 上腹部,脐中上5寸,前正中线旁开2寸。

主治 胃痛,腹胀,呕吐,食欲不振。

Location:5 cun above the umbilicus,2 cun lateral to the anterior midline.

Indications:gastric pain,abdominal distension,vomiting,poor appetite.

ST21 梁门 LiángMén

位置　上腹部,脐中上 4 寸,前正中线旁开 2 寸。

主治　胃痛,呕吐,食欲不振,腹胀,泄泻。

Location：4 cun above the umbilicus, 2 cun lateral to the anterior midline.

Indications：gastric pain, vomiting, poor appetite, abdominal distension, diarrhea.

ST22 关门 GuānMén

位置　上腹部,脐中上 3 寸,前正中线旁开 2 寸。

主治　腹胀,腹痛,食欲不振,肠鸣泄泻,水肿。

Location：3 cun above the umbilicus, 2 cun lateral to the anterior midline.

Indications：abdominal distension or pain, poor appetite, borborygmus, diarrhea, edema.

ST23 太乙 TàiYǐ

位置　上腹部,脐中上 2 寸,前正中线旁开 2 寸。

主治　胃痛,心烦,癫狂。

Location：2 cun above the umbilicus, 2 cun lateral to the anterior midline.

Indications：gastric pain, irritability, mental disorder.

ST24 滑肉门 HuáRòuMén

位置　上腹部,脐中上 1 寸,前正中线旁开 2 寸。

主治　胃痛,呕吐,癫狂。

Location：1 cun above the umbilicus, 2 cun lateral to the anterior midline.

Indications：gastric pain, vomiting, mental disorder.

ST25 天枢 TiānShū (大肠募穴)

位置　腹部,横平脐中,前正中线旁开 2 寸。

主治　腹痛,腹胀,肠鸣,绕脐痛,便秘,泄泻,痢疾,月经不调,水肿。

Location：2 cun lateral to the centre of umbilicus.

Indications：abdominal pain or distension, borborygmus, constipation, diarrhea, dysentery, irregular menstruation, edema.

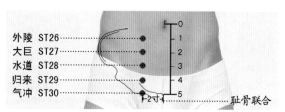

外陵 ST26
大巨 ST27
水道 ST28
归来 ST29
气冲 ST30

耻骨联合

ST26 外陵 WàiLíng

位置　下腹部,脐中下1寸,前正中线旁开2寸。

主治　腹痛,疝气,痛经。

Location：in the lower abdomen，1 cun below the umbilicus，2 cun lateral to the anterior midline.

Indications：abdominal pain，hernia，dysmenorrhea.

ST27 大巨 DàJù

位置　下腹部,脐中下2寸,前正中线旁开2寸。

主治　小腹胀满,小便不利,疝气,遗精,早泄。

Location：2 cun below the umbilicus，2 cun lateral to the anterior midline.

Indications：lower abdominal distension，urination disturbance，hernia，semInal emission，ejaculatio praecox.

ST28 水道 ShuǐDào

位置　下腹部,脐中下3寸,前正中线旁开2寸。

主治　小腹胀满,小便不通,水肿,疝气,痛经,不孕。

Location：3 cun below the umbilicus，2 cun lateral to the anterior midline.

Indications：lower abdominal distension，retention of urine，edema，hernia，dysmenorrhea，infertility.

ST29 归来 GuīLái

位置　下腹部,脐中下4寸,前正中线旁开2寸。

主治　小腹痛,疝气,月经不调,闭经,带下,阴挺。

Location：4 cun below the umbilicus，2 cun lateral to the anterior midline.

Indications: abdominal pain, hernia, dysmenorrhea, irregular menstruation, amenorrhea, morbid leukorrhea, prolapse of uterus.

ST30 气冲 QìChōng

位置 腹股沟区,耻骨联合上缘,前正中线旁开 2 寸,动脉搏动处。

主治 腹痛肠鸣,疝气,外阴肿痛,阳痿,月经不调。

Location: in the inguinal groove, at the upper border of the symphysis pubis, 2 cun lateral to the anterior midline, at where th femoral artery beats.

Indications: abdominal pain, borborygmus, hernia, pain and swelling of external genitalia, impotence, irregular menstruation.

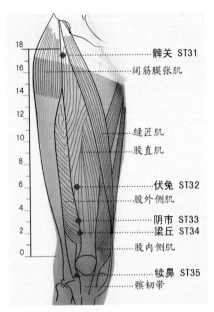

ST31 髀关 BìGuān

位置 股前区,股直肌近端、缝匠肌与阔筋膜张肌3条肌肉之间凹陷中。

主治 腰膝冷痛,下肢无力。

Location: in the anterior aspect of thigh, in the depression between the proximal end of rectus femoris, m. Sartorius and tensor fasciae

Indications: cold pain in the lumbar and knees, weakness of the lower limbs.

ST32 伏兔 FúTù

位置 股前区,髌底上6寸,髂前上棘与髌底外侧端的连线上。

主治 下肢瘫痪,麻痹,膝关节炎,脚气。

Location: 6 cun above the laterosuperior border of patella, in the line connecting the anterior superior iliac spine and lateral border of patella.

Indications: paralysis, numbness or pain of the lower limbs, gonitis, beriberi.

ST33 阴市 YīnShì

位置　股前区,髌底上 3 寸,股直肌肌腱外侧缘。

主治　腿膝麻痹、疼痛,屈伸不利。

Location: 3 cun above the laterosuperior border of patella, in the lateral side of the tendon of m. rectus femoris.

Indications: numbness, pain or motor impairment of lower limbs and knee.

ST34 梁丘 LiángQiū (郄穴)

位置　股前区,髌底上 2 寸,股外侧肌与股直肌肌腱之间。

主治　膝胫痹痛,胃痛,乳痈,下肢不遂。

Location: 2 cun above the laterosuperior border of patella, between the tendons of m. vastus lateralis and m. rectus femoris.

Indications: pain and swelling of the knee and leg, gastric pain, mastitis, motor impairment of the lower limbs.

ST35 犊鼻 DúBí

位置　膝前区,髌韧带外侧凹陷中。

主治　膝痛,麻木,屈伸不利。

Location: in the depression lateral to the patellar ligament.

Indications: pain, numbness or motor impairment of the knee.

ST

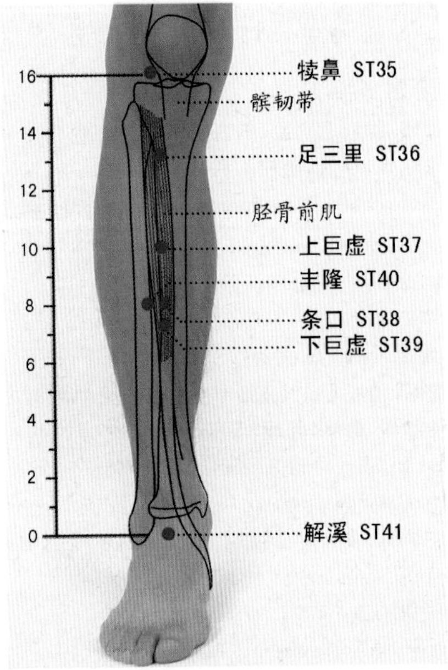
犊鼻 ST35
髌韧带
足三里 ST36
胫骨前肌
上巨虚 ST37
丰隆 ST40
条口 ST38
下巨虚 ST39
解溪 ST41
16
14
12
10
8
6
4
2
0

ST36 足三里 ZúSānLǐ（合穴；胃腑下合穴）

位置 小腿外侧，犊鼻（ST35）下 3 寸，犊鼻（ST35）与解溪（ST41）连线上。

主治 胃痛，呕吐，呃逆，腹胀，肠鸣，泄泻，痢疾，便秘，乳痈，肠痈，膝胫疼痛，脚气，水肿，咳嗽，气喘，虚劳羸瘦，疳积，完谷不化，中风，瘫痪，头晕，失眠，癫狂。

Location: 3 cun below DúBí (ST35), in the line connecting DúBí (ST35) and JiěXī (ST41).

Indications: gastric pain, vomiting, hiccup, abdominal distension, borborygmus, diarrhea, dysentery, constipation, mastitis, enteritis, pain of the knee joint and leg, beriberi, edema, apcough, asthma, emaciation due to general deficiency, indigestion, apoplexy, hemiplegia, dizziness, insomnia, mental disorder.

ST37 上巨虚 ShàngJùXū (大肠腑下合穴)

位置　小腿外侧,犊鼻(ST35)下 6 寸,犊鼻(ST35)与解溪(ST41)连线上。

主治　腹痛,腹胀,肠鸣,泄泻,痢疾,便秘,肠痈,中风瘫痪。

Location: 6 cun below DúBí (ST35), in the line connecting DúBí (ST35) and JiěXī (ST41).

Indications: abdominal pain or distension, borborygmus, diarrhea, dysentery, constipation, enteritis, paralysis due to stroke.

ST38 条口 TiáoKǒu

位置　小腿外侧,犊鼻(ST35)下 8 寸,犊鼻(ST35)与解溪(ST41)连线上。

主治　膝胫麻木、疼痛,足缓不收,肩痛不举,脘腹疼痛。

Location: 8 cun below Dúbí (ST35), in the line connecting DúBí (ST35) and JiěXī (ST41).

Indications: numbness, or pain of the knee and leg, weakness and motor impairment of the foot, pain, motor impairment of the shoulder, epigastric or abdominal pain.

ST39 下巨虚 XiàJùXū (小肠腑下合穴)

位置　小腿外侧,犊鼻(ST35)下 9 寸,犊鼻(ST35)与解溪(ST41)连线上。

主治　小腹痛,腰背痛引睾丸,乳痈,下肢痿痹。

Location: 9cun below DúBí (ST35), in the line connecting DúBí (ST35) and JiěXī (ST41).

Indications: lower abdominal pain, back pain referring to the testis, mastitis, muscular atrophy or pain of the lower limbs.

ST40 丰隆 FēngLóng (络穴)

位置　小腿外侧,外踝尖上8寸,胫骨前肌的外缘。

主治　头痛,眩晕,咳嗽,哮喘,痰多,胸痛,便秘,癫狂,痫证,下肢痿痹、肿痛。

Location: 8 cun superior to the tip of the external malleolus, lateral to the anterior border of the tibia.

Indications: headache, dizziness, vertigo, cough, asthma, excessive sputum, chest pain, constipation, mental disorder, epilepsy, muscular atrophy, pain, swelling or paralysis of the lower limbs.

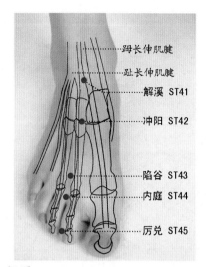

姆长伸肌腱

趾长伸肌腱

解溪 ST41

冲阳 ST42

陷谷 ST43

内庭 ST44

厉兑 ST45

ST41 解溪 JiěXī (经穴)

位置 踝区,踝关节前面中央凹陷中,姆长伸肌腱与趾长伸肌腱之间。

主治 踝关节疼痛,下肢痿痹,癫狂,头痛,眩晕,腹胀,便秘。

Location:in the ankle, at the midpoint of the transverse crease of the ankle joint, between the tendons of m. extensor digitorum longus and hallucis longus.

Indications:ankle pain, muscular atrophy or pain of the lower limbs, epilepsy, headache,dizziness, vertigo, abdominal distension, constipation.

ST42 冲阳 ChōngYáng (原穴)

位置 足背,第2跖骨基底部与中间楔状骨关节处,可触及足背动脉。

主治 上齿痛,足背红肿,口眼歪斜,足痿。

Location:in the dorsum of foot, between the base of the second metatarsal bone and the cuneiform bone, where the pulsation of the dorsal artery of foot is palpable.

Indications:Pain of the upper teeth, redness and swelling of the dorsum of foot, facial paralysis, muscular atrophy and motor impairment of the foot.

ST43 陷谷 XiànGǔ (输穴)

位置　足背,第2、3跖骨间,第2跖趾关节近端凹陷中。

主治　面浮,身肿,腹痛,肠鸣,足背肿痛。

Location：in the depression proximal to the junction of the second and third metatarsal bones.

Indications：facial or general edema, abdominal pain, borborygmus, swelling and pain in the dorsum of foot.

ST44 内庭 NèiTíng (荥穴)

位置　足背,第2、3趾骨间,趾蹼缘后方赤白肉际处。

主治　齿痛,面痛,鼻衄,胃痛,吐酸,腹胀,泄泻,便秘,足背肿痛,热病。

Location：proximal to the web margin between the second and third toes, at the junction of the red and white skin.

Indications：toothache, trigeminal neuralgia, epistaxis, gastric pain, acid regurgitation, abdominal distension, diarrhea, constipation, swelling and pain in the dorsum of foot, febrile diseases.

ST45 厉兑 LìDuì (井穴)

位置　足趾,第2趾末节外侧,趾甲根角侧后方0.1寸(指寸)。

主治　面肿,鼻衄,口角歪斜,齿痛,喉痹,腹胀,足胫寒冷,热病,多梦,癫狂。

Location：in the lateral side of the terminal phalanx of the second toe, 0.1 cun from the corner of nail.

Indications：facial swelling, deviation of the mouth, toothache, sore throat, loss of voice, abdominal distension, cold sensation in the leg and foot, dream-disturbed sleep, mental disorder.

4. 足太阴脾经 Spleen Meridian of Foot Taiyin

足太阴脾经分寸歌

大趾内侧端隐白，节前陷中求大都。

太白节后白肉际，节后一寸公孙呼。

商丘踝前陷中有，踝上三寸三阴交。

踝上六寸漏谷是，膝下五寸地机朝。

膝下内侧阴陵泉，血海膝膑上内廉。

箕门穴在鱼腹取，动脉应手越筋间。

冲门横骨两端同，去腹中行三寸半。

冲上七分是府舍，舍上三寸腹结算。

结上三寸是大横，去与脐平莫的乱。

建里这旁四寸取，便是腹哀分一段。

中庭旁六食窦穴，膻中去六是天溪。

再上寸六胸乡穴，周荣相去亦同稽。

大包腋下有六寸，渊腋之下三寸分。

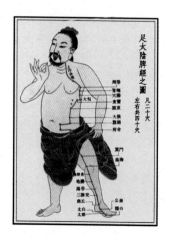

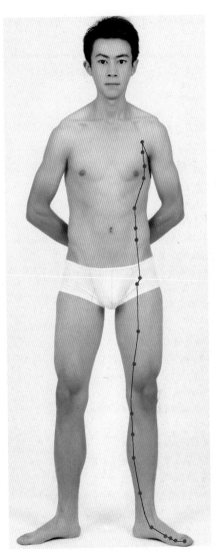

足太阴脾经

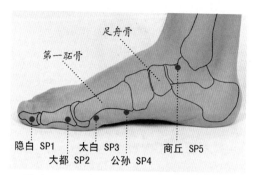

隐白 SP1　太白 SP3　　商丘 SP5
大都 SP2　公孙 SP4

SP1 隐白 YīnBái (井穴)

位置　足趾,大趾末节内侧,趾甲根角侧后方0.1寸(指寸)。

主治　腹胀,崩漏,癫狂,多梦,惊风。

Location：in the medial side of the terminal phalanx of the big toe, 0.1 cun from the corner of nail.

Indications：abdominal distension, uterine bleeding, mental disorder, dream-disturbed sleep, convulsion.

SP2 大都 DàDū (荥穴)

位置　足趾,第1跖趾关节远端赤白肉际凹陷中。

主治　腹胀,胃痛,热病无汗。

Location：in the medial side of the big toe, distal to the first metatarsophalangeal joint, in the depression at the junction of the red and white skin.

Indications：abdominal distension, gastric pain, febrile diseases with anhidrosis.

SP3 太白 TàiBái (输、原穴)

位置　跖区,第1跖趾关节近端赤白肉际凹陷中。

主治　胃痛,腹胀,便秘,痢疾,吐泻,身重,脚气。

Location：proximal to the 1st metatarsophalangeal joint, in the depression at the junction of the red and white skin.

Indications：gastric pain, abdominal distension, constipation, dysentery, vomiting, diarrhea, heavy sensation of the body, beriberi.

SP4 公孙 GōngSūn(络穴、八脉交会穴)

位置 跖区,第1跖骨底的前下缘赤白肉际处。

主治 胃痛,呕吐,腹胀,泄泻,痢疾。

Location:in the depression distal and inferior to the base of the first metatarsal bone, at the junction of the red and white skin.

Indications:gastric pain, vomiting, abdominal distension, diarrhea, dysentery.

SP5 商丘 ShāngQiū(经穴)

位置 踝区,内踝前下方,舟骨粗隆与内踝尖连线的中点凹陷中。

主治 腹胀,便秘,泄泻,肠鸣,舌本强痛,足踝痛。

Location:in the depression distal and inferior to the medial malleolus, midway between the tuberosity of the navicular bone and the tip of the medial malleolus.

Indications:abdominal distension, constipation, diarrhea, borborygmus, pain and rigidity of the tongue, pain in the foot and ankle.

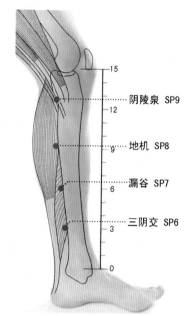

阴陵泉 SP9

地机 SP8

漏谷 SP7

三阴交 SP6

SP6 三阴交 SānYīnJiāo

位置 小腿内侧,内踝尖上3寸,胫骨内侧缘后际。

主治 腹痛,肠鸣,腹胀,泄泻,月经不调,带下,阴挺,遗精,遗尿,下肢痿痹,失眠。

Location:3 cun directly above the tip of the medial malleolus, posterior to the medial border of the tibia.

Indications:abdominal pain, borborygmus, abdominal distension, diarrhea, irregular menstruation, morbid leukorrhea, prolapse of uterus, nocturnal emission, enuresis, muscular atrophy, motor impairment, paralysis or pain of the lower limbs, insomnia.

SP7 漏谷 LòuGǔ

位置 小腿内侧,内踝尖上6寸,胫骨内侧缘后际。

主治 腹胀,肠鸣,腿膝厥冷、麻痹。

Location: 6 cun above the tip of the medial malleolus, posterior to the medial border of the tibia.

Indications: abdominal distension, borborygmus, coldness, numbness or paralysis of the knee and leg.

SP8 地机 DìJī(郄穴)

位置 小腿内侧,阴陵泉(SP9)下 3 寸,胫骨内侧缘后际。

主治 腹痛,腹胀,泄泻,水肿,小便不利,遗精,月经不调,痛经。

Location: 3 cun below YīnLíngQuán (SP9), posterior to the medial border of the tibia.

Indications: abdominal pain or distension, diarrhea, edema, urination disturbance, nocturnal emission, irregular menstruation, dysmenorrhea.

SP9 阴陵泉 YīnLíngQuán(合穴)

位置 小腿内侧,胫骨内侧髁下缘与胫骨内侧缘之间的凹陷中。

主治 腹痛,腹胀,泄泻,痢疾,水肿,黄疸,小便不利,遗尿,尿失禁,阴部痛,痛经,膝痛。

Location: in the depression between the lower border of the medial condyle of the tibia and the medial border of the tibia.

Indications: abdominal pain or distension, diarrhea, dysentery, edema, jaundice, urination disturbance, enuresis, incontinence of urine, pain in the external genitalia, dysmenorrhea, knee pain.

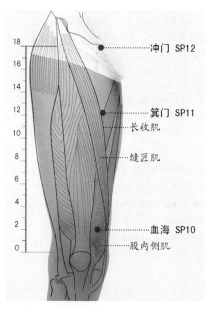

SP10 血海 XuèHǎi

位置 股前区,髌底内侧端上 2 寸,股内侧肌隆起处。

主治 月经不调,痛经,崩漏,闭经,风疹,湿疹,股内侧痛。

Location: in the anterior aspect of the thigh, 2 cun above the mediosuperior border of the patella, at the prominence of the vastus medialis.

Indications: irregular menstruation, dysmenorrhea, uterine bleeding, amenorrhea, urticaria, eczema, pain in the medial aspect of the thigh.

SP11 箕门 JīMén

位置 股前区,髌底内侧端与冲门(SP12)的连线上 1/3 与下 2/3 交点,长收肌和缝匠肌交角的动脉搏动处。

主治 小便不利,遗尿,腹股沟肿痛,下肢痿痹。

Location: in the anterior aspect of the thigh, at the junction of the upper one-third and lower two-thirds in the line connecting the medioinferior end of the patella and ChōngMén (SP12), at the pulsation of the artery in the angle formed by the adductor longus and musculus sartorius.

Indications: urination disturbance, enuresis, pain and swelling in the inguinal region, muscular atrophy, motor impairment, pain and paralysis of the lower limbs.

SP12 冲门 ChōngMén

位置　腹股沟区,腹股沟斜纹中,髂外动脉搏动处的外侧。

主治　腹痛,疝气,小便不利。

Location: superior to the lateral end of the inguinal groove, lateral to the pulsating external iliac artery.

Indications: abdominal pain, hernia, urination disturbance.

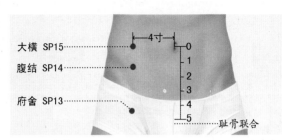

大横 SP15 ....

腹结 SP14 ....

府舍 SP13 ....

├─4寸─┤

0
1
2
3
4
5

耻骨联合

SP13 府舍 FǔShě

位置 下腹部,脐中下4.3寸,前正中线旁开4寸。

主治 少腹痛,疝气。

Location：4 cun below the umbilicus, 4 cun lateral to the anterior midline.

Indications：pain in the sides of lower abdomen, hernia.

SP14 腹结 FùJié

位置 下腹部,脐中下1.3寸,前正中线旁开4寸。

主治 绕脐腹痛,腹胀,疝气,泄泻,便秘。

Location：1.3 cun below the umbilicus, 4 cun lateral to the anterior midline.

Indications：pain around the umbilical region, abdominal distension, hernia, diarrhea, constipation.

SP15 大横 DàHéng

位置 腹部,脐中旁开4寸。

主治 腹痛,腹胀,泄泻,痢疾,大便秘结。

Location：4 cun lateral to the centre of the umbilicus.

Indications：abdominal pain or distension, diarrhea, dysentery, constipation.

天溪 SP18
食窦 SP17
腹哀 SP16

SP16 腹哀 Fù'āi

位置 上腹部,脐中上3寸,前正中线旁开4寸。

主治 腹痛,完谷不化,便秘,痢疾。

Location:3 cun above the centre of the umbilicus,4 cun lateral to the anterior midline.

Indications:abdominal pain,indigestion,constipation,dysentery.

SP17 食窦 ShíDòu

位置 胸部,第5肋间隙,前正中线旁开6寸。

主治 胸胁胀痛。

Location:in the fifth intercostal space,6 cun lateral to the anterior midline.

Indications:distending pain in the chest and hypochondriac region.

SP18 天溪 TiānXī

位置 胸部,第4肋间隙,前正中线旁开6寸。

主治 胸胁胀痛,咳嗽,乳痈,乳汁少。

Location:in the fourth intercostal space,6 cun lateral to the anterior midline.

Indications:distending pain in the chest and hypochondrium,cough,mastitis,insufficient lactation.

周荣 SP20

胸乡 SP19

4 3 2 1 0 1 2 3 4

大包 SP21

SP19 胸乡 XiōngXiāng

位置 胸部,第 3 肋间隙,前正中线旁开 6 寸。

主治 胸胁胀痛。

Location：in the third intercostal space，6 cun lateral to the anterior midline.

Indications：distending pain in the chest and hypochondrium.

SP20 周荣 ZhōuRóng

位置 胸部,第 2 肋间隙,前正中线旁开 6 寸。

主治 胸胁胀满,咳嗽气逆。

Location：in the second intercostal space，6 cun lateral to the anterior midline.

Indications：fullness in the chest and hypochondriac region，cough，hiccup.

SP21 大包 DàBāo(脾之大络穴)

位置 胸外侧区,第 6 肋间隙,在腋中线上。

主治 胸胁痛,气喘,全身疼痛,四肢无力。

Location：in the lateral side of the chest，in the 6th intercostal space，at the middle axillary line.

Indications：pain in the chest and hypochondriac region，asthma，general pain and weakness.

5. 手少阴心经 Heart Meridian of Hand Shaoyin

手少阴心经分寸歌

少阴心经极泉中,腋下筋间动引胸。
青灵肘上三寸觅,少海肘后五分通。
灵道掌后一寸半,通里腕后一寸同。
阴郄去腕五分在,神门掌后锐骨逢。
少府小指本节末,小指内侧是少冲。

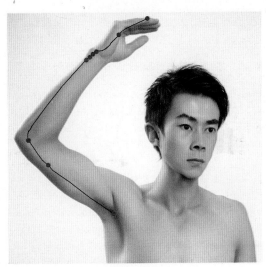

手少阴心经

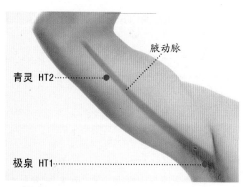

腋动脉

青灵 HT2

极泉 HT1

HT1 极泉 JíQuán

位置 腋区,腋窝中央,腋动脉搏动处。

主治 心痛,胁肋痛,瘰疬,肘臂冷痛。

Location：in the centre of the axilla, at the pulsation of the axillary artery.

Indications：pain in the costal and cardiac regions, scrofula, cold pain of the elbow and arm.

HT2 青灵 QīngLíng

位置 臂前区,肘横纹上3寸,肱二头肌内侧沟中。

主治 心痛,胁痛,肩臂痛。

Location：3 cun above the medial end of the transverse cubital crease, in the groove medial to m. biceps brachii.

Indications：pain in the cardiac and hypochondriac regions, shoulder and arm.

HT3 少海 ShàoHǎi(合穴)

位置 肘前区,横平肘横纹,肱骨内上髁前缘。

主治 心痛,手臂挛痛,麻木,手颤,瘰疬,腋胁痛。

Location：at the level of the transverse cubital crease, in the upper border of the medial epicondyle of humerus.

Indications：cardiac pain, spasmodic pain or numbness of the hand and arm, tremor of the hand, scrofula, pain in the axilla and hypochondriac region.

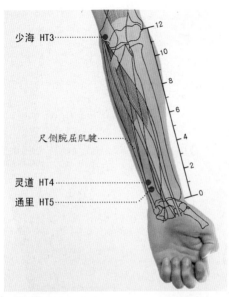

少海 HT3

尺侧腕屈肌腱

灵道 HT4
通里 HT5

HT4 灵道 LíngDào (经穴)

位置　前臂前区,腕掌侧远端横纹上1.5寸,尺侧腕屈肌腱桡侧缘。

主治　心痛,肘臂挛痛,暴喑。

Location：in the palmar aspect of the forearm, 1.5 cun above the distal transverse crease of the wrist, at the radial side of the tendon of m. flexor carpi radialis.

Indications：cardiac pain, spasmodic pain of the elbow and arm, sudden loss of voice.

HT5 通里 TōngLǐ (络穴)

位置　前臂前区,腕掌侧远端横纹上1寸,尺侧腕屈肌腱桡侧缘。

主治　心悸,怔忡,头晕,目眩,咽喉肿痛,暴喑,舌强不语,腕臂痛。

Location：in the palmar aspect of the forearm, 1 cun above the distal transverse crease of the wrist, at the radial side of the tendon of m. flexor carpi radialis.

Indications：palpitation, vertigo, dizziness, sore throat, sudden loss of voice, aphasia with stiffness of the tongue, pain in the wrist and elbow.

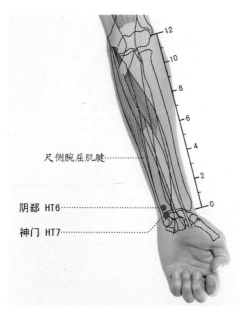

尺侧腕屈肌腱············

阴郄 HT6 ············

神门 HT7 ············

HT6 阴郄 YīnXì(郄穴)

位置　前臂前区,腕掌侧远端横纹上 0.5 寸,尺侧腕屈肌腱的桡侧缘。

主治　心痛,惊悸,骨蒸盗汗,吐血,衄血,暴喑。

Location：in the palmar aspect of the forearm, 0.5 cun above the distal transverse crease of the wrist, on the radial side of the tendon of m. flexor carpi radialis.

Indications：cardiac pain, palpitation, night sweating, hematemesis, epistaxis, sudden loss of voice.

HT7 神门 ShénMén(输穴、原穴)

位置　腕前区,腕掌侧远端横纹尺侧端,尺侧腕屈肌腱的桡侧缘。

主治　心痛,心烦,怔忡,惊悸,健忘,失眠,癫狂,胁痛,掌中热,目黄。

Location：in the ulnar end of the distal transverse crease of the wrist, at the radial side of the tendon of m. flexor carpi radialis.

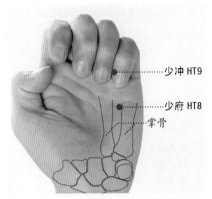

少冲 HT9

少府 HT8

掌骨

Indications：cardiac pain, irritability, palpitation, poor memory, insomnia, mental disorder, pain in the hypochondriac region, feverish sensation in the palm, yellow sclera.

HT8 少府 ShàoFǔ(荥穴)

位置　手掌,横平第5掌指关节近端,第4、5掌骨之间。

主治　心悸,胸痛,小指挛痛,掌中热,遗尿,小便不利,阴痒。

Location：in the palm, at the level of the proximal part of the fifth metacarpophalangeal joint, between the fourth and fifth metacarpal bones.

Indications：palpitation, chest pain, spasmodic pain of the little finger, hot sensation in the palm, enuresis, urination disturbance, pruritus vulvae.

HT9 少冲 ShàoChōng(井穴)

位置　手指,小指末节桡侧,指甲根角侧上方0.1寸(指寸)。

主治　心悸,心痛,胸胁痛,癫狂,热病,昏厥。

Location：in the radial side of the terminal phalanx of the little finger, 0.1 cun from the corner of nail.

Indications：palpitation, cardiac pain, pain in the chest and hypochondriac regions, mental disorder, febrile diseases, loss of consciousness.

6. 手太阳小肠经 Small Intestine Meridian of Hand Taiyang

手太阳小肠经分寸歌

小指端外少泽明，前谷外侧节后觅。
节后握拳取后溪，腕骨腕前骨陷侧。
锐骨下陷阳谷找，腕后锐上觅养老。
支正腕后五寸量，小海肘后五分好。
肩贞胛下两筋解，臑俞大骨下陷保。
天宗秉风后骨中，秉风臑外举有空。
曲垣肩中曲肩陷，外俞去脊三寸从。
中俞二寸大椎旁，天窗扶突后陷详。
天容耳下曲颊后，颧髎面頄锐端量。
听宫耳中大如菽，此上小肠手太阳。

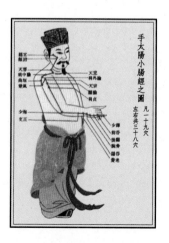

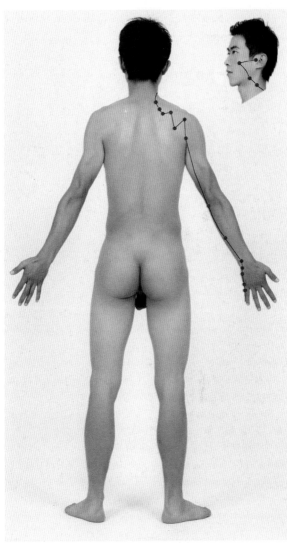

手太阳小肠经

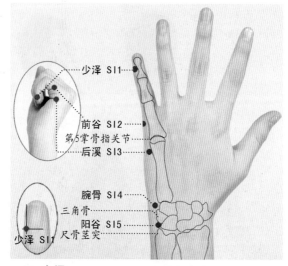

少泽 SI1
前谷 SI2
第5掌骨指关节
后溪 SI3
腕骨 SI4
三角骨
阳谷 SI5
少泽 SI1 尺骨茎突

SI1 少泽 ShàoZé(井穴)

位置　手指,小指末节尺侧,指甲根角侧上方0.1寸(指寸)。

主治　头痛,热病,昏厥,乳汁少,咽喉肿痛,目赤,目翳。

Location：on the ulnar side of the little finger, 0. 1 cun from the corner of nail.

Indications：headache, febrile diseases, loss of consciousness, insufficient lactation, sore throat, red eyes, cloudiness of the cornea.

SI2 前谷 QiánGǔ(荥穴)

位置　手指,第5掌指关节尺侧远端赤白肉际凹陷中。

主治　手指麻木,热病,耳鸣,头痛,小便赤。

Location：in the finger, on the ulna side of the crease distal to the fifth metacarpophalangeal joint, at the junction of the red and white skin.

Indications：numbness of the fingers, febrile disease, tinnitus, headache, deep yellow urine.

SI3 后溪 HòuXī(输穴、八脉交会穴)

位置 手内侧,第 5 掌指关节尺侧近端赤白肉际凹陷中。

主治 头项强痛,耳鸣,耳聋,咽喉肿痛,癫狂,疟疾,闪腰,盗汗,热病,手指挛急,麻木,肩臂疼痛。

Location: on the ulna side of the crease proximal to the fifth metacarpophalangeal joint, at the junction of the red and white skin.

Indications: pain and rigidity of the neck, tinnitus, deafness, sore throat, mental disorder, malaria, acute lumbar sprain, night sweating, febrile diseases, spasm or numbness of the fingers, pain in the shoulder and arm.

SI4 腕骨 WànGǔ(原穴)

位置 腕区,第 5 掌骨基底与三角骨之间的赤白肉际凹陷中。

主治 热病无汗,头痛,项强,指挛腕痛,黄疸。

Location: on the ulna side of the palm, in the depression between the base of the fifth metacarpal bone and the triangular bone.

Indications: febrile diseases with anhidrosis, headache, neck rigidity, spasm of the fingers, jaundice.

SI5 阳谷 YángGǔ(经穴)

位置 腕后区,尺骨茎突与三角骨之间的凹陷中。

主治 颈颌肿,手腕痛,热病。

Location: in the depression between the styloid process of the ulna and the triangular bone.

Indications: swelling of the neck and mandibular region, pain of the hand and wrist, febrile diseases.

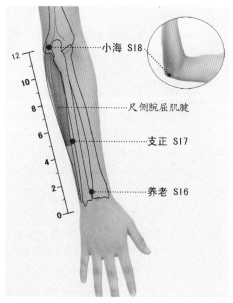

小海 SI8

尺侧腕屈肌腱

支正 SI7

养老 SI6

SI6 养老 YǎngLǎo(郄穴)

位置　前臂后区,腕背横纹上1寸,尺骨头桡侧凹陷中。

主治　目视不明,肘、肩、臂疼痛。

Location：1 cun above the dorsal crease of the wrist, in the depression on the radial side of the styloid process of the ulna.

Indications：blurred vision, pain in the elbow, arm or shoulder.

SI7 支正 ZhīZhèng(络穴)

位置　前臂后区,腕背侧远端横纹上5寸,尺骨尺侧与尺侧腕屈肌之间。

主治　项强,头痛,目眩,肘臂,手指挛痛,热病,癫狂。

Location：5 cun proximal to the dorsal crease of the wrist, between the ulna border of the ulna and the flexor carpi ulnaris.

Indications：neck rigidity, headache, dizziness, spasmodic pain in the elbow and fingers, febrile diseases, mental disorder.

SI8 小海 XiǎoHǎi（合穴）

位置　肘后区,尺骨鹰嘴与肱骨内上髁之间凹陷中。

主治　头痛,癫痫,齿龈炎,肘臂外后侧痛。

Location：in the depression between the olecranon of the ulna and the medial epicondyle of the humerus.

Indications：headache, epilepsy, swelling of the cheek, pain in the lateroposterior aspect of the elbow and arm.

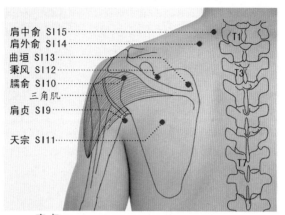

SI9 肩贞 JiānZhēn

位置 肩胛区，肩关节后下方，腋后纹头直上 1 寸。

主治 肩胛痛，手臂不举。

Location: in the scapular region, posterior and inferior to the shoulder joint, 1 cun above the posterior end of the axillary fold.

Indications: pain in the scapular region, motor impairment of the hand and arm.

SI10 臑俞 NàoShū

位置 肩胛区，腋后纹头直上，肩胛冈下缘凹陷中。

主治 肩肿，肩臂酸痛无力。

Location: in the scapular region, directly above the end of the posterior axillary fold, in the depression inferior to the scapular spine.

Indications: swelling of the shoulder, pain and weakness of the shoulder and arm.

SI11 天宗 TiānZōng

位置 肩胛区，肩胛冈中点与肩胛骨下角连线上 1/3 与下 2/3 交点凹陷中。

主治 肩胛痛，肘臂外后侧痛。

Location: in the scapula, in the depression at the junction of the upper one-third and lower two-thirds of the line connecting the midpoint of scapular spine and the inferior angle of scapula.

Indications: pain in the scapular region, pain in the lateroposterior aspect of the elbow and arm.

SI12 秉风 BǐngFēng

位置　肩胛区,肩胛冈中点上方冈上窝中。

主治　肩胛痛,上肢酸麻,肩臂不举。

Location: in the center of the suprascapular fossa.

Indications: pain in the scapular region, numbness or pain of the upper limbs, motor impairment of the shoulder and arm.

SI13 曲垣 QūYuán

位置　肩胛区,肩胛冈内侧端上缘凹陷中。

主治　肩胛拘急疼痛。

Location: in the scapular region, in the depression at the medial extremity of the suprascapular fossa.

Indications: pain and stiffness in the scapular region.

SI14 肩外俞 JiānWàiShū

位置　脊柱区,第1胸椎棘突下,后正中线旁开3寸。

主治　肩背疼痛,颈项强痛。

Location: in the vertebral column area, at the level of the lower border of the spinous process of the first thoracic vertebra, 3 cun lateral to the posterior midline.

Indications: pain of the shoulder and back, pain and rigidity of the neck.

SI15 肩中俞 JiānZhōngShū

位置　脊柱区,第7颈椎棘突下,后正中线旁开2寸。

主治　咳嗽,气喘,肩背疼痛。

Location: in the vertebral column area, at the level of the lower border of the spinous process of the seventh cervical vertebra, 2 cun lateral to the posterior midline.

Indications: cough, asthma, pain of the shoulder and back.

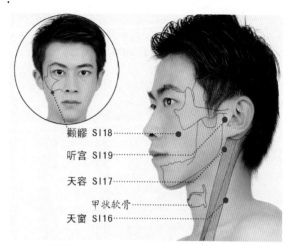

颧髎 SI18

听宫 SI19

天容 SI17

甲状软骨

天窗 SI16

SI16 天窗 TiānChuāng

位置 颈部,横平喉结,胸锁乳突肌的后缘。

主治 咽喉肿痛,暴喑,耳聋,耳鸣,颈项强痛。

Location：in the neck，at the level of the prominentia laryngea，at the posterior border of m. sternocleidomastoideus.

Indications：sore throat，sudden loss of voice，deafness，tinnitus，stiffness and pain of the neck.

SI17 天容 TiānRóng

位置 颈部,下颌角后方,胸锁乳突肌的前缘凹陷中。

主治 耳聋,耳鸣,咽喉肿痛,颊肿,咽中如梗,瘿气。

Location：in the neck，posterior to the angle of mandible，in the depression at the anterior border of m. sternocleidomastoideus.

Indications：deafness，tinnitus，sore throat，swelling of the cheek，foreign body sensation in the throat，goiter.

SI18 颧髎 QuánLiáo

位置 面部,颧骨下缘,目外眦直下凹陷中。

主治 口眼歪斜,眼睑眴动,面痛,齿痛,颊肿,目黄。

Location：in the face，at the lower border of zygoma，in the depression directly below the outer canthus.

Indications: facial paralysis, twitching of eyelids, pain in the face, toothache, swelling of the cheek, yellow sclera.

SI19 听宫 TīngGōng

位置 面部,耳屏正中与下颌骨髁突之间的凹陷中。

主治 耳鸣,耳聋,聤耳,齿痛。

Location: in the face, in the depression between the tragus and the condyloid process of the mandible.

Indications: tinnitus, deafness, otorrhea, toothache.

7. 足太阳膀胱经 Bladder Meridian of Foot Taiyang

足太阳膀胱经分寸歌

足太阳属膀胱经，目内眦角始睛明。
眉毛内侧攒竹取，眉冲直上旁神庭。
曲差入发五分际，神庭旁开寸五分。
五处旁开亦寸半，故与上星穴相平。
承光通天络却穴，相去寸半调匀看。
玉枕夹脑一寸三，入发三寸枕骨安。
天柱项后平哑门，大筋外廉陷中存。
自此夹脊开寸五，第一大杼二风门。
三椎肺俞四厥阴，心五督六膈下会。
膈七肝九十胆俞，十一脾俞十二胃。
十三三焦十四肾，气海俞在十五椎。
大肠十六椎下取，十七关元俞可推。
小肠十八胱十九，中膂俞穴二十随。
白环廿一椎下是，上下分寸细推量。
更有上次中下髎，一二三四腰空好。
会阳阴毛尻骨旁，第一侧线穴尽考。
继向臀部横纹取，承扶居下陷中央。
殷门扶下方六寸，浮郄系居委阳上。
委阳腘外两筋乡，相去中有一寸长。
委中在腘横纹里，向上另起一排行。
第二侧线三寸旁，第二椎下附分裹。
三椎魄户四膏肓，第五椎下寻神堂。
第六譩譆膈关七，第九魂门十阳纲。

十一椎下为意舍,十二胃仓穴细商。
十三肓门端正在,十四志室切莫忘。
十九胞肓廿一秩,委下二寸寻合阳。
承筋合阳直下取,穴在腨肠之中藏。
承山腨下分肉间,外踝七寸上飞扬。
跗阳外踝上三寸,昆仑后跟陷中详。
仆参跟下脚边上,申脉踝下五分张。
金门申前墟后取,京骨外侧骨际量。
束骨本节后肉际,通谷节前陷中乡。
至阴却在小趾侧,取剌从其甲角旁。

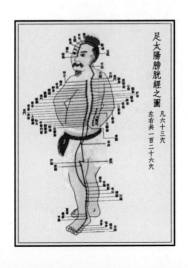

足太陽膀胱經之圖

凡六十三穴
左右共一百二十六穴

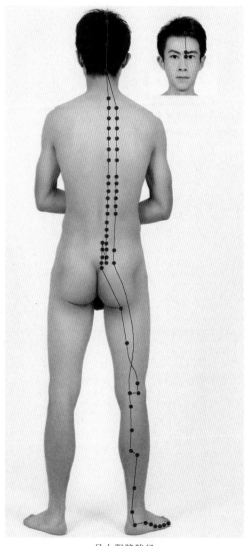

足太阳膀胱经

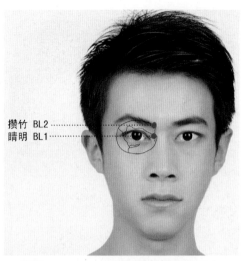

攒竹 BL2
睛明 BL1

BL1 睛明 JīngMíng

位置 面部,目内眦内上方眶内侧壁凹陷中。

主治 目赤肿痛,眦痒,迎风流泪,夜盲,色盲,目眩,近视。

Location: in the face, in the depression at the orbital medial wall mediosuperior to the inner canthus.

Indications: redness, swelling and pain of the eye, itching of the canthus, lacrimation induced by wind, night blindness, colour blindness, blurred vision, myopia.

BL2 攒竹 CuánZhú

位置 面部,眉头凹陷中,额切迹处。

主治 头痛,目眩,眉棱骨痛,目视不明,迎风流泪,目赤肿痛,眼睑瞤动,青盲。

Location: at the medial extremity of the eyebrow, or the supra-orbital notch.

Indications: headache, blurred vision, pain in the supraorbital region, lacrimation induced by wind, redness, swelling and pain of the eye, twitching of eyelids, glaucoma.

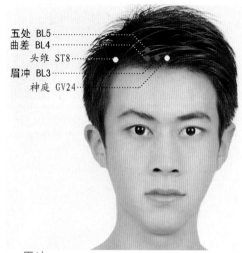

五处 BL5
曲差 BL4
头维 ST8
眉冲 BL3
神庭 GV24

BL3 眉冲 MéiChōng

位置 头部，额切迹直上入发际0.5寸。

主治 头痛，眩晕，痫证。

Location: in the head, directly above the supraorbital notch, 0.5 cun within the anterior hairline.

Indications: headache, dizziness, vertigo, epilepsy.

BL4 曲差 QǔChā

位置 头部，前发际正中直上0.5寸，旁开1.5寸。

主治 头痛，鼻塞，鼻衄，目视不明，目眩。

Location: 0.5cun directly above the midpoint of the anterior hairline and 1.5 cun lateral to the midline.

Indications: headache, nasal obstruction, epistaxis, blurred vision.

BL5 五处 WǔChù

位置 头部，前发际正中直上1寸，旁开1.5寸。

主治 头痛，目眩，痫证。

Location: 1 cun directly above the midpoint of the anterior hairline and 1.5 cun lateral to the midline.

Indications: headache, blurred vision, epilepsy.

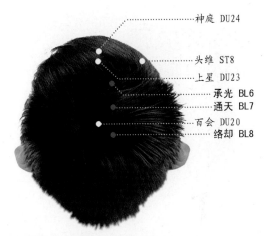

神庭 DU24

头维 ST8
上星 DU23
承光 BL6
通天 BL7
百会 DU20
络却 BL8

BL6 承光 ChéngGuāng

位置　头部，前发际正中直上 2.5 寸，旁开 1.5 寸。

主治　头痛，目眩，鼻塞。

Location：2.5 cun directly above the midpoint of the anterior hairline and 1.5 cun lateral to the midline.

Indications：headache, blurred vision, nasal obstruction.

BL7 通天 TōngTiān

位置　头部，前发际正中直上 4 寸，旁开 1.5 寸。

主治　头痛，眩晕，鼻塞，鼻衄，鼻渊。

Location：4 cun directly above the midpoint of the anterior hairline and 1.5 cun lateral to the midline.

Indications：headache, dizziness, vertigo, nasal obstruction, epistaxis, rhinorrhea.

BL8 络却 LuòQuè

位置　头部，前发际正中直上 5.5 寸，旁开 1.5 寸。

主治　眩晕，目视不明，耳鸣，癫狂。

Location：5.5 cun directly above the midpoint of the anterior hairline and 1.5 cun lateral to the midline.

Indications：dizziness, vertigo, blurred vision, tinnitus, mental disorder.

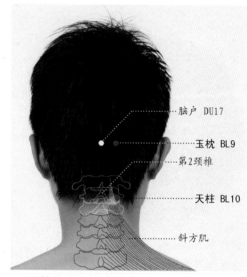

脑户 DU17

玉枕 BL9

第2颈椎

天柱 BL10

斜方肌

BL

BL9 玉枕 YùZhěn

位置 头部,横平枕外隆凸上缘,后发际正中旁开1.3寸。

主治 头项痛,眩晕,目痛,鼻塞。

Location: at the level of the upper border of the external occipital protuberance, 1.3 cun lateral to the midpoint of the posterior hairline.

Indications: headache, neck pain, dizziness, vertigo, ophthalmalgia, nasal obstruction.

BL10 天柱 TiānZhù

位置 颈后区,横平第2颈椎棘突上际,斜方肌外缘凹陷中。

主治 头痛,鼻塞,咽喉肿痛,项强,肩背痛。

Location: at the level of the second cervical vertebra, in the depression on the lateral aspect of m. trapezius.

Indications: Headache, nasal obstruction, sore throat, neck rigidity, pain in the shoulder and back.

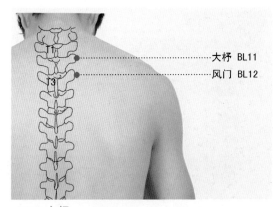

大杼 BL11

风门 BL12

BL11 大杼 DàZhù(骨会穴)

位置 脊柱区,第1胸椎棘突下,后正中线旁开1.5寸。

主治 头痛,项背痛,肩胛疼痛,咳嗽,发热,颈项强直。

Location: in the vertebral column area, at the level of the lower border of the spinous process of the first thoracic vertebra, 1.5 cun lateral to the posterior midline.

Indications: headache, pain in the neck or back, pain and soreness in the scapular region, cough, fever, neck rigidity.

BL12 风门 FēngMén

位置 脊柱区,第2胸椎棘突下,后正中线旁开1.5寸。

主治 咳嗽,发热,头痛,项强。

Location: at the level of the lower border of the spinous process of the second thoracic vertebra, 1.5 cun lateral to the posterior midline.

Indications: cough, fever, headache, neck rigidity.

BL

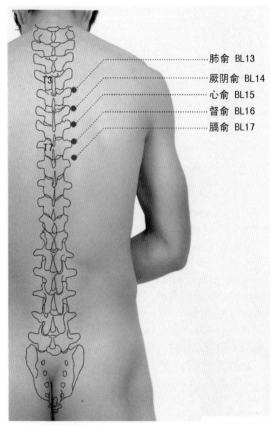

肺俞 BL13
厥阴俞 BL14
心俞 BL15
督俞 BL16
膈俞 BL17

BL13 肺俞 FèiShū(背俞穴)

位置 脊柱区,第 3 胸椎棘突下,后正中线旁开 1.5 寸。

主治 咳嗽,气喘,胸痛,吐血,骨蒸潮热,盗汗。

Location:at the level of the lower border of the spinous process of the third thoracic vertebra, 1.5 cun lateral to the posterior midline.

Indications:cough, asthma, chest pain, hematemesis, afternoon fever, night sweating.

BL14 厥阴俞 JuéYīnShū (背俞穴)

位置 脊柱区，第 4 胸椎棘突下，后正中线旁开 1.5 寸。

主治 咳嗽，心痛，心悸，胸闷，呕吐。

Location: at the level of the lower border of the spinous process of the fourth thoracic vertebra, 1.5 cun lateral to the posterior midline.

Indications: cough, cardiac pain, palpitation, oppressing feeling in the chest, vomiting.

BL15 心俞 XīnShū (背俞穴)

位置 脊柱区，第 5 胸椎棘突下，后正中线旁开 1.5 寸。

主治 心痛，惊悸，健忘，心烦，咳嗽，吐血，梦遗，盗汗，癫狂，痫证。

Location: at the level of the lower border of the spinous process of the fifth thoracic vertebra, 1.5 cun lateral to the posterior midline.

Indications: cardiac pain, palpitation, poor memory, irritability, cough, hematemesis, nocturnal emission, night sweating, mental disorder, epilepsy.

BL16 督俞 DūShū

位置 脊柱区，第 6 胸椎棘突下，后正中线旁开 1.5 寸。

主治 心痛，胃痛。

Location: at the level of the lower border of the spinous process of the sixth thoracic vertebra, 1.5 cun lateral to the posterior midline.

Indications: cardiac pain, gastric pain.

BL17 膈俞 GéShū (血会穴)

位置 脊柱区，第 7 胸椎棘突下，后正中线旁开 1.5 寸。

主治 呕吐，呃逆，噎膈，饮食不下，气喘，咳嗽，吐血，潮热，盗汗，风疹。

Location: at the level of the lower border of the spinous process of the seventh thoracic vertebra, 1.5 cun lateral to the posterior midline.

Indications: vomiting, hiccup, belching, dysphagia, asthma, cough, hematemesis, afternoon fever, night sweating, measles.

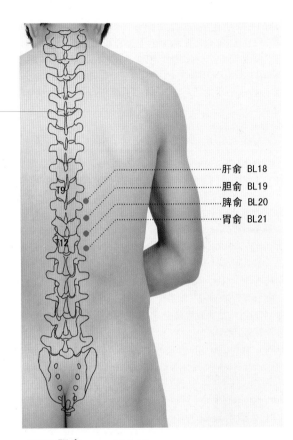

肝俞 BL18

胆俞 BL19

脾俞 BL20

胃俞 BL21

BL18 肝俞 GānShū(背俞穴)

位置 脊柱区,第 9 胸椎棘突下,后正中线旁开 1.5 寸。

主治 黄疸,胁痛,目赤,目眩,夜盲,癫狂,痫症,脊背痛,吐血,鼻衄。

Location: at the level of the lower border of the spinous process of the ninth thoracic vertebra, 1.5 cun lateral to the posterior midline.

Indications: jaundice, pain in the hypochondriac region, redness of the eye, blurred vision, night blindness, mental disorder, epilepsy, back pain, hematemesis, epistaxis.

BL19 胆俞 DǎnShū(背俞穴)

位置 脊柱区,第 10 胸椎棘突下,后正中线旁开 1.5 寸。

主治 黄疸,口苦,胸胁痛,肺痨,潮热。

Location: at the level of the lower border of the spinous process of the tenth thoracic vertebra, 1.5 cun lateral to the posterior midline.

Indications: jaundice, bitter taste in the mouth, pain in the chest and hypochondriac region, pulmonary tuberculosis, afternoon fever.

BL20 脾俞 PíShū(背俞穴)

位置 脊柱区,第 11 胸椎棘突下,后正中线旁开 1.5 寸。

主治 胃脘痛,腹胀,呕吐,泄泻,便血,月经过多,水肿,背痛。

Location: at the level of the lower border of the spinous process of the eleventh thoracic vertebra, 1.5 cun lateral to the posterior midline.

Indications: epigastric pain, abdominal distension, vomiting, diarrhea, hematochezia, profuse menstruation, edema, back pain.

BL21 胃俞 WèiShū(背俞穴)

位置 脊柱区,第 12 胸椎棘突下,后正中线旁开 1.5 寸。

主治 胸胁痛,胃脘痛,纳呆,腹胀,肠鸣,泄泻,呕吐。

Location: at the level of the lower border of the spinous process of the twelfth thoracic vertebra, 1.5 cun lateral to the posterior midline.

Indications: pain in the chest, hypochondrium or epigastrium, poor appetite, abdominal distension, borborygmus, diarrhea, vomiting.

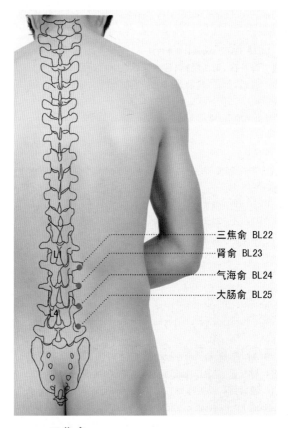

三焦俞 BL22
肾俞 BL23
气海俞 BL24
大肠俞 BL25

BL22 三焦俞 SānJiāoShū(背俞穴)

位置　脊柱区,第1腰椎棘突下,后正中线旁开1.5寸。

主治　腹胀,肠鸣,完谷不化,呕吐,泄泻,痢疾,水肿,腰背强痛。

Location：at the level of the lower border of the spinous process of the first lumbar vertebra, 1.5 cun lateral to the posterior midline.

Indications：abdominal distension, borborygmus, indigestion, vomiting, diarrhea, dysentery, edema, pain and stiffness of the low back.

BL23 肾俞 ShènShū(背俞穴)

位置 脊柱区,第 2 腰椎棘突下,后正中线旁开 1.5 寸。

主治 遗精,阳痿,月经不调,腰膝酸软,头昏目眩,耳鸣,耳聋,水肿,气喘。

Location: at the level of the lower border of the spinous process of the second lumbar vertebra, 1.5 cun lateral to the posterior midline.

Indications: nocturnal emission, impotence, enuresis, irregular menstruation, lumbago, weakness of the knee, blurred vision, dizziness, tinnitus, deafness, edema, asthma, diarrhea.

BL24 气海俞 QìHǎiShū

位置 脊柱区,第 3 腰椎棘突下,后正中线旁开 1.5 寸。

主治 腰痛,月经不调,痛经,气喘。

Location: at the level of the lower border of the spinous process of the third lumbar vertebra, 1.5 cun lateral to the posterior midline.

Indications: lumbago, irregular menstruation, dysmenorrhea, asthma.

BL25 大肠俞 DàChángShū(背俞穴)

位置 脊柱区,第 4 腰椎棘突下,后正中线旁开 1.5 寸。

主治 腰背疼痛,腹胀,肠鸣,泄泻,便秘,下肢痿痹,腰腿痛。

Location: at the level of the lower border of the spinous process of the fourth lumbar vertebra, 1.5 cun lateral to the posterior midline.

Indications: lumbago, abdominal distension, borborygmus, diarrhea, constipation, muscular atrophy, pain, numbness or motor impairment of the lower limbs, sciatica.

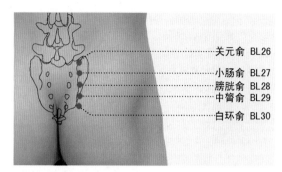

关元俞 BL26
小肠俞 BL27
膀胱俞 BL28
中膂俞 BL29
白环俞 BL30

BL26 关元俞 GuānYuánShū

位置 脊柱区,第5腰椎棘突下,后正中线旁开1.5寸。

主治 腰痛,腹胀,泄泻,遗尿,腰腿痛,小便频数。

Location：at the level of the lower border of the spinous process of the fifth lumbar vertebra, 1.5 cun lateral to the posterior midline.

Indications：lumbago, abdominal distension, diarrhea, enuresis, sciatica, frequency of urination.

BL27 小肠俞 XiǎoChángShū(背俞穴)

位置 骶区,横平第1骶后孔,骶正中嵴旁开1.5寸。

主治 小腹胀痛,痢疾,遗精,尿血,遗尿,白带,腰骶痛,腰腿痛。

Location：in the sacrum, at the level of the first posterior sacral foramen, 1.5 cun lateral to the median sacral crest.

Indications：lower abdominal pain or distension, dysentery, nocturnal emission, hematuria, enuresis, morbid leukorrhea, lumbosacral pain, sciatica.

BL28 膀胱俞 PángGuāngShū(背俞穴)

位置 骶区,横平第2骶后孔,骶正中嵴旁开1.5寸。

主治 小便不通,遗尿,尿频,泄泻,便秘,腰背强痛。

Location：at the level of the second posterior sacral foramen, 1.5 cun lateral to the median sacral crest.

Indications：retention to urine, enuresis, frequency of urination, diarrhea, constipation, stiffness and pain of the low back.

BL29 中膂俞 ZhōngLǚShū

位置　骶区，横平第 3 骶后孔，骶正中嵴旁开 1.5 寸。

主治　痢疾，疝气，腰背强痛。

Location: at the level of the third posterior sacral foramen, 1.5 cun lateral to the median sacral crest.

Indications: dysentery, hernia, stiffness and pain of the low back.

BL30 白环俞 BáiHuánShū

位置　骶区，横平第 4 骶后孔，骶正中嵴旁开 1.5 寸。

主治　遗尿，疝痛，白带，月经不调，腰髋冷痛，二便不利，里急后重，脱肛。

Location: at the level of the fourth posterior sacral foramen, 1.5 cun lateral to the median sacral crest.

Indications: enuresis, pain due to hernia, morbid leukorrhea, irregular menstruation, cold sensation and pain of the low back, urination disturbance, constipation, tenesmus, prolapse of rectum.

BL

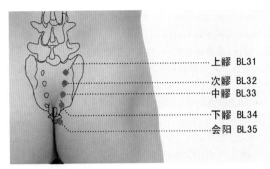

上髎 BL31
次髎 BL32
中髎 BL33
下髎 BL34
会阳 BL35

BL31 上髎 ShàngLiáo

位置　骶区,正对第 1 骶后孔中。

主治　腰痛,二便不利,月经不调,赤白带下,阴挺。

Location:in the sacrum, at the first posterior sacral foramen

Indications: lumbago, urination disturbance, constipation, irregular menstruation, morbid leukorrhea, prolapse of uterus.

BL32 次髎 CìLiáo

位置　骶区,正对第 2 骶后孔中。

主治　腰痛,疝气,月经不调,遗精,阳痿,遗尿,小便不利,下肢痿痹。

Location: in the sacrum, at the second posterior sacral foramen.

Indications: lumbago, hernia, irregular menstruation, nocturnal emission, impotence, enuresis, urination disturbance, muscular atrophy, pain, numbness and motor impairment of the lower limbs.

BL33 中髎 ZhōngLiáo

位置　骶区,正对第 3 骶后孔中。

主治　腰痛,便秘,泄泻,小便不利,月经不调,带下。

Location: in the sacrum, at the third posterior sacral foramen.

Indications: lumbago, constipation, diarrhea, urination disturbance, irregular menstruation, morbid leukorrhea.

BL34 下髎 XiàLiáo

位置　骶区，正对第 4 骶后孔中。

主治　腰痛，小腹痛，小便不利，便秘，带下。

Location: in the sacrum, at the fourth posterior sacral foramen.

Indications: lumbago, lower abdominal pain, urination disturbance, constipation, morbid leukorrhea.

BL35 会阳 HuìYáng

位置　骶区，尾骨端旁开 0.5 寸。

主治　痢疾，便血，泄泻，痔疾，阳痿，带下。

Location: in the sacrum, 0.5 cun lateral to the tip of the coccyx.

Indications: dysentery, hematochezia, diarrhea, hemorrhoids, impotence, morbid leucorrhea.

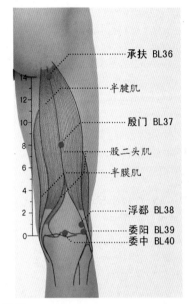

承扶 BL36

半腱肌

殷门 BL37

股二头肌

半膜肌

浮郄 BL38

委阳 BL39

委中 BL40

BL36 承扶 ChéngFú

位置 股后区,臀沟的中点。

主治 腰骶臀股疼痛,下肢痿痹,大便难,痔疾。

Location: in the posterior aspect of the thigh, at the midpoint of the inferior gluteal crease.

Indications: pain in the lumbosacral and gluteal regions, muscular atrophy, pain, numbness and motor impairment of the lower limbs, constipation, hemorrhoids.

BL37 殷门 YīnMén

位置 股后区,臀沟下6寸,股二头肌与半腱肌之间。

主治 腰痛,腰腿痛,下肢痿痹,瘫痪。

Location: in the posterior aspect of the thigh, 6 cun below the inferior gluteal crease, between the biceps femoris and semitendinosus.

Indications: lumbago, sciatica, muscular atrophy, pain, numbness or motor impairment of the lower limbs, hemiplegia.

BL38 浮郄 FúXì

位置　膝后区,腘横纹上1寸,股二头肌腱的内侧缘。

注:稍屈膝,委阳(BL39)上1寸,股二头肌腱的内侧缘。

主治　臀股麻木。

Location: in the posterior aspect of the thigh, 1 cun above the WěiYáng(BL39), at the medial side of the tendon of m. biceps femoris.

Indications: numbness of the gluteal and femoral regions.

BL39 委阳 WěiYáng(三焦腑下合穴)

位置　膝部,腘横纹上,股二头肌腱的内侧缘。

主治　腰背强痛,小腹胀满,水肿,小便不利,腿足挛痛。

Location: in the knee, at the transverse crease of the popliteal fossa, in the medial border of the tendon of m. biceps femoris.

Indications: stiffness and pain of the low back, distension and fullness of the lower abdomen, edema, urination disturbance, cramp of the leg and foot.

BL40 委中 WěiZhōng(合穴)

位置　膝后区,腘横纹中点。

主治　腰痛,髋关节活动不利,下肢痿痹,半身不遂,腹痛,吐泻。

Location: in the posterior side of the knee, at the midpoint of the transverse crease of the popliteal fossa.

Indications: lumbago, motor impairment of the hip joint, muscular atrophy, pain, motor impairment of the lower limbs, hemiplegia, abdominal pain, vomiting, diarrhea.

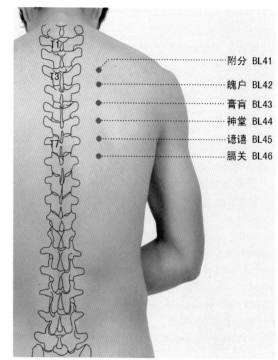

附分 BL41
魄户 BL42
膏肓 BL43
神堂 BL44
谚谑 BL45
膈关 BL46

BL41 附分 FùFēn

位置 脊柱区,第 2 胸椎棘突下,后正中线旁开 3 寸。

主治 肩背拘急,颈项强痛,肘臂麻木。

Location：in the vertebral column area, at the level of the lower border of the spinous process of the second thoracic vertebra, 3 cun lateral to the posterior midline.

Indications：stiffness and pain of the shoulder, back and neck, numbness of the elbow and arm.

BL42 魄户 PòHù

位置 脊柱区,第 3 胸椎棘突下,后正中线旁开 3 寸。

主治 肺痨,咳血,咳嗽,气喘,项强,肩背痛。

Location：at the level of the lower border of the spinous process of the third thoracic vertebra, 3 cun lateral to the posterior midline.

Indications: pulmonary tuberculosis, hemoptysis, cough, asthma, neck rigidity, pain in the shoulder and back.

BL43 膏肓 GāoHuāng

位置　脊柱区,第 4 胸椎棘突下,后正中线旁开 3 寸。

主治　肺痨,咳嗽,气喘,吐血,盗汗,健忘,遗精。

Location: at the level of the lower border of the spinous process of the fourth thoracic vertebra, 3 cun lateral to the posterior midline.

Indications: pulmonary tuberculosis, cough, asthma, hematemesis, night sweating, poor memory, nocturnal emission.

BL44 神堂 ShénTáng

位置　脊柱区,第 5 胸椎棘突下,后正中线旁开 3 寸。

主治　气喘,心痛,心悸,胸闷,咳嗽,脊背强痛。

Location: at the level of the lower border of the spinous process of the fifth thoracic vertebra, 3 cun lateral to the posterior midline.

Indications: asthma, cardiac pain, palpitation, oppressing feeling in the chest, cough, stiffness and pain of the back.

BL45 譩譆 YìXǐ

位置　脊柱区,第 6 胸椎棘突下,后正中线旁开 3 寸。

主治　咳嗽,气喘,肩背痛。

Location: at the level of the lower border of the spinous process of the sixth thoracic vertebra, 3 cun lateral to the posterior midline.

Indications: cough, asthma, pain of the shoulder and back.

BL46 膈关 GéGuān

位置　脊柱区,第 7 胸椎棘突下,后正中线旁开 3 寸。

主治　饮食不下,呃逆,呕吐,嗳气,脊背强痛。

Location: at the level of the lower border of the spinous process of the seventh thoracic vertebra, 3 cun lateral to the posterior midline.

Indications: dysphagia, hiccup, vomiting, belching, pain and stiffness of the back.

BL

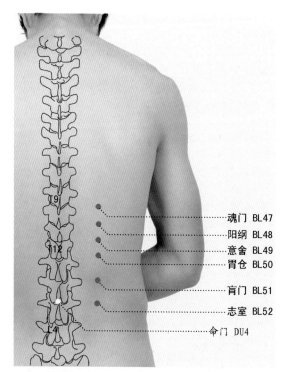

魂门 BL47
阳纲 BL48
意舍 BL49
胃仓 BL50
肓门 BL51
志室 BL52
命门 DU4

BL47 魂门 HúnMén

位置 脊柱区,第 9 胸椎棘突下,后正中线旁开 3 寸。

主治 胸胁痛,背痛,呕吐,泄泻。

Location：at the level of the lower border of the spinous process of the ninth thoracic vertebra，3 cun lateral to the posterior midline.

Indications：pain in the chest and hypochondriac region，back pain，vomiting，diarrhea.

BL48 阳纲 YángGāng

位置 脊柱区,第 10 胸椎棘突下,后正中线旁开 3 寸。

主治 肠鸣,腹痛,泄泻,胁痛,黄疸。

Location: at the level of the lower border of the spinous process of the tenth thoracic vertebra, 3 cun lateral to the posterior midline.

Indications: borborygmus, abdominal pain, diarrhea, pain in the hypochondriac region, jaundice.

BL49 意舍 YìShè

位置 脊柱区，第 11 胸椎棘突下，后正中线旁开 3 寸。

主治 腹胀，肠鸣，呕吐，泄泻，饮食不下。

Location: at the level of the lower border of the spinous process of the eleventh thoracic vertebra, 3 cun lateral to the posterior midline.

Indications: abdominal distension, borborygmus, vomiting, diarrhea, dysphagia.

BL50 胃仓 WèiCāng

位置 脊柱区，第 12 胸椎棘突下，后正中线旁开 3 寸。

主治 腹胀，胃脘痛，脊背痛，小儿食积。

Location: at the level of the lower border of the spinous process of the twelfth thoracic vertebra, 3 cun lateral to the posterior midline.

Indications: abdominal distension, pain in the epigastric region and back, infantile indigestion.

BL51 肓门 HuāngMén

位置 腰区，第 1 腰椎棘突下，后正中线旁开 3 寸。

主治 腹痛，便秘，痞块。

Location: at the level of the lower border of the spinous process of the first lumbar vertebra, 3 cun lateral to the posterior midline.

Indications: abdominal pain, constipation, abdominal mass.

BL52 志室 ZhìShì

位置 腰区，第 2 腰椎棘突下，后正中线旁开 3 寸。

主治 肠鸣，腹胀，腰背痛，小便不利，遗精，阳痿。

Location: at the level of the lower border of the spinous process of the second lumbar vertebra, 3 cun lateral to the posterior midline.

Indications: borborygmus, abdominal distension, pain in the low back, urination disturbance, nocturnal emission, impotence.

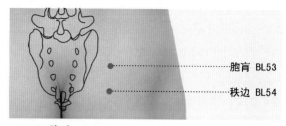

胞肓 BL53

秩边 BL54

BL53 胞肓 BāoHuāng

位置　骶区,横平第 2 骶后孔,骶正中嵴旁开 3 寸。

主治　肠鸣,腹胀,腰背痛。

Location：in the sacrum, at the level of the second sacral posterior foramen, 3 cun lateral to the median sacral crest.

Indications：borborygmus, abdominal distension, pain in the low back.

BL54 秩边 ZhìBiān

位置　骶区,横平第 4 骶后孔,骶正中嵴旁开 3 寸。

主治　腰骶痛,下肢痿痹,小便不利,痔疾,大便难。

Location：at the level of the fourth posterior sacral foramen, 3 cun lateral to the median sacral crest.

Indications：pain in the lumbosacral region, muscular atrophy or motor impairment of the lower limbs, urination disturbance, hemorrhoids, constipation.

BL

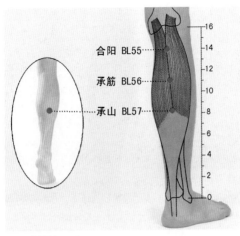

BL55 合阳 HéYáng

位置　小腿后区,腘横纹下 2 寸,腓肠肌内、外侧头之间。

主治　腰背痛,下肢酸痛、麻痹。

Location：in the posterior aspect of the leg, 2 cun below the transverse crease of the popliteal fossa, between the medial and lateral heads of m. gastrocnemius.

Indications：lumbago, pain or paralysis of the lower limbs.

BL56 承筋 ChéngJīn

位置　小腿后区,腘横纹下 5 寸,腓肠肌两肌腹之间。

主治　腿痛转筋,痔疾,腰背拘急。

Location：5 cun below the transverse crease of the popliteal fossa, between the two bellies of m. gastrocnemius.

Indications：spasm of the gastrocnemius, hemorrhoids, acute low back pain.

BL57 承山 ChéngShān

位置　小腿后区,腓肠肌两肌腹与肌腱交角处。

主治　腰痛,腿痛转筋,痔疾,便秘。

Location：in a pointed depression formed below the gastrocnemius muscle belly.

Indications：lumbago, spasm of the gastrocnemius, hemorrhoids, constipation.

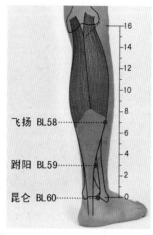

飞扬 BL58
跗阳 BL59
昆仑 BL60

BL58 飞扬 FēiYáng（络穴）

位置　小腿后区,昆仑(BL60)直上 7 寸,腓肠肌外下缘与跟腱移行处。

主治　头痛,目眩,鼻塞,鼻衄,腰背痛,痔疾,腿软无力。

Location：7 cun directly above KūnLún（BL60）, between the lateroinferior border of m. gastrocnemius and tendo calcaneus.

Indications：headache, vertigo, nasal obstruction, epistaxis, back pain, hemorrhoids, weakness of the leg.

BL59 跗阳 FūYáng（阳跷脉郄穴）

位置　小腿后区,昆仑(BL60)直上 3 寸,腓骨与跟腱之间。

主治　头重,头痛,腰骶痛,外踝肿痛,下肢瘫痪。

Location：3 cun directly above KūnLún（BL60）, between the fibula and tendo calcaneus.

Indications：heavy sensation of the head, headache, pain in the lumbosacral region, swelling and pain of the external malleolus, paralysis of the lower limbs.

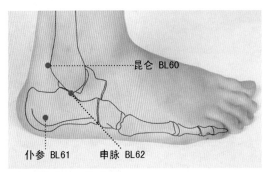

昆仑 BL60

仆参 BL61　　申脉 BL62

BL60 昆仑 KūnLún (经穴)

位置　踝区,外踝尖与跟腱之间的凹陷中。

主治　头痛,目眩,项强,鼻衄,肩背腰腿痛,脚跟肿痛,难产,痫证。

Location: in the depression between the tip of the external malleolus and tendo calcaneus.

Indications: headache, vertigo, neck rigidity, epistaxis, pain in the shoulder, back and arm, swelling and pain of the heel, difficult labour, epilepsy.

BL61 仆参 PúCān

位置　跟区,昆仑(BL60)直下,跟骨外侧,赤白肉际处。

主治　下肢痿痹,足跟痛。

Location: directly below KūnLún (BL60), lateral to the calcaneus, at the junction of the red and white skin.

Indications: muscular atrophy or pain of the lower limbs, pain in the heel.

BL62 申脉 ShēnMài (八脉交会穴)

位置　踝区,外踝尖直下,外踝下缘与跟骨之间凹陷中。

主治　痫症,癫狂,头痛,眩晕,失眠,腰腿疼痛。

Location: directly below the tip of external malleolus, in the depression between the inferior border of the external malleolus and the calcaneus.

Indications: epilepsy, mental disorder, headache, dizziness, vertigo, insomnia, back pain, pain of the leg.

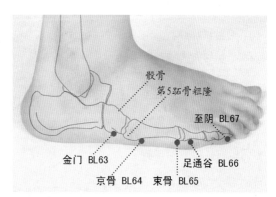

骰骨
第5跖骨粗隆
至阴 BL67
金门 BL63
京骨 BL64 束骨 BL65
足通谷 BL66

BL63 金门 JīnMén(郄穴)

位置 足背,外踝前缘直下,第5跖骨粗隆后方,骰骨下缘凹陷中。

主治 癫狂,痫证,小儿惊风,腰痛,外踝痛,下肢痹痛。

Location: directly below the anterior border of the external malleolus, proximal to the tuberosity of the fifth metatarsal bone, in the depression of the inferior border of the cuboid bone.

Indications: mental disorder, epilepsy, infantile convulsion, back pain, pain in the external malleolus, motor impairment and pain of the lower limbs.

BL64 京骨 JīngGǔ(原穴)

位置 跖区,第5跖骨粗隆前下方,赤白肉际处。

主治 头痛,项强,腰腿痛,痫证。

Location: distal and inferior to the tuberosity of the fifth metatarsal bone, at the junction of the red and white skin.

Indications: headache, neck rigidity, pain in the lumbar and thigh, epilepsy.

BL65 束骨 ShùGǔ(输穴)

位置 跖区,第5跖趾关节的近端,赤白肉际处。

主治 癫狂,头痛,项强,目眩,腰背及下肢后侧痛。

Location: proximal to the fifth metatarsophalangeal joint, at the junction of the red and white skin.

BL

Indications: mental disorder, headache, neck rigidity, vertigo, back pain, pain in lateral aspect of the lower limbs.

BL66 足通谷 ZúTōngGǔ(荥穴)

位置　足趾,第5跖趾关节的远端,赤白肉际处。

主治　头痛,项强,目眩,鼻衄,癫狂。

Location: distal to the fifth metatarsophalangeal joint, at the junction of the red and white skin.

Indications: headache, neck rigidity, vertigo, epistaxis, mental disorder.

BL67 至阴 ZhiYīn(井穴)

位置　足趾,小趾末节外侧,趾甲跟角侧后方0.1寸(指寸)。

主治　头痛,鼻塞,鼻衄,目痛,胎位不正,难产,胞衣不下。

Location: in the lateral side of the terminal phalanx of the little toe, 0.1 cun from the corner of nail.

Indications: headache, nasal obstruction, epistaxis, ophthalmalgia, malposition of fetus, difficult labour, retention of placenta.

BL

8. 足少阴肾经 Kidney Meridian of Foot Shaoyin

足少阴肾经分寸歌

足掌心中是涌泉，然谷踝前大骨边。

太溪踝后跟骨上，照海踝下四分安。

水泉溪下一寸觅，大钟跟后踵筋间。

复溜溪上二寸取，交信溜前五分骈。

二穴只隔筋前后，太阴之后少阴前。

筑宾处腨上腨分，阴谷膝下内辅边。

上从任脉开半寸，横骨平取曲骨边。

大赫气穴并四满，中注肓俞亦相连。

六穴上行皆一寸，俱距中行半寸间。

商曲又平下脘取，石关阴都通谷联。

幽门适当巨阙侧，五穴分寸量同前。

再从中行开二寸，步廊却在中庭边。

神封灵墟及神藏，彧中俞府璇玑旁。

每穴上行皆寸六，旁开二寸仔细量。

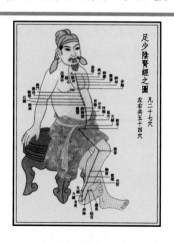

足少阴肾经之图

凡二十七穴

左右共五十四穴

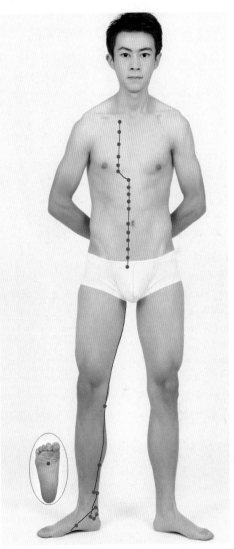

足少阴肾经

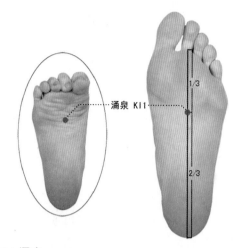

涌泉 KI1

KI1 涌泉 YǒngQuán(井穴)

位置 足底,屈足卷趾时足心最凹陷中。

主治 头痛,目眩,头昏,咽喉痛,舌干,失音,大便难,小便不利,小儿惊风,足心热,昏厥。

Location:in the sole, in the depression when the foot is in plantar flexion.

Indications:headache, blurred vision, dizziness, sore throat, dryness of the tongue, loss of voice, constipation, urination disturbance, infantile convulsions, feverish sensation in the sole, loss of consciousness.

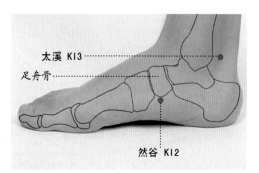

太溪 KI3
足舟骨
然谷 KI2

KI2 然谷 RánGǔ(荥穴)

位置 足内侧,足舟骨粗隆下方,赤白肉际处。

主治 阴痒,阴挺,月经不调,遗精,咳血,消渴,泄泻,足背肿痛,小儿脐风。

Location: inferior to the tuberosity of the navicular bone, at the junction of the red and white skin.

Indications: pruritus vulvae, prolapse of uterus, irregular menstruation, nocturnal emission, hemoptysis, diabetes, diarrhea, swelling and pain of the dorsum of foot, acute infantile omphalitis.

KI3 太溪 TàiXī(输穴,原穴)

位置 踝区,内踝尖与跟腱之间的凹陷中。

主治 咽喉干痛,齿痛,耳聋,耳鸣,头晕,咳血,气喘,消渴,月经不调,失眠,遗精,阳痿,小便频数,腰背痛。

Location: in the depression between the tip of the medial malleolus and tendo calcaneus.

Indications: sore throat, toothache, deafness, tinnitus, dizziness, hematemesis, asthma, diabetes, irregular menstruation, insomnia, nocturnal emission, impotence, frequency of urination, lumbago.

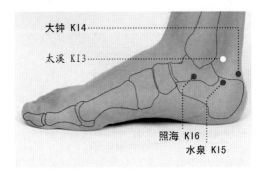

KI4 大钟 DàZhōng(络穴)

位置　跟区,内踝后下方,跟骨上缘,跟腱附着部前缘凹陷中。

主治　咳血,气喘,腰背强痛,二便不利,足跟痛。

Location：posterior and inferior to the medial malleolus, at the upper border of calcaneus, in the depression anterior to the medial said of the attachment of tendo calcaneus.

Indications：hematemesis, asthma, stiffness and pain of the low back, urination disturbance, constipation, pain in the heel.

KI5 水泉 ShuiQuán(郄穴)

位置　跟区,太溪(KI3)直下 1 寸,跟骨结节内侧凹陷中。

主治　闭经,月经不调,痛经,阴挺,小便不利。

Location：1 cun directly below TàiXī (KI3), in the depression at the medial side of the tuberosity of the calcaneum.

Indications：amenorrhea, irregular menstruation, dysmenorrhea, prolapse of uterus, urination disturbance.

KI6 照海 ZhàoHǎi(八脉交会穴)

位置　踝区,内踝尖下 1 寸,内踝下缘边际凹陷中。

主治　月经不调,赤白带下,阴挺,阴痒,小便频数,癃闭,便秘,痫证,失眠,咽喉干痛,气喘。

Location: 1 cun below the tip of the medial malleolus, in the depression below the tip of the medial malleolus.

Indications: irregular menstruation, morbid leukorrhea, prolapse of uterus, pruritus vulvae, frequency of urination, retention of urine, constipation, epilepsy, insomnia, sore throat, asthma.

K I

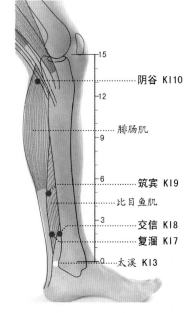

阴谷 KI10

腓肠肌

筑宾 KI9

比目鱼肌

交信 KI8

复溜 KI7

太溪 KI3

KI7 复溜 FùLiū(经穴)

位置 小腿内侧,内踝尖上 2 寸,跟腱的前缘。

主治 水肿,腹胀,泄泻,肠鸣,足痿,盗汗,自汗,热病汗不出。

Location：in the medial aspect of the leg, 2 cun directly above the tip of the external malleolus, at the anterior border of tendo calcaneus.

Indications：edema, abdominal distension, diarrhea, borborygmus, muscular atrophy of the leg, night sweating, spontaneous sweating, febrile diseases without sweating.

KI8 交信 JiāoXìn(阴跷脉郄穴)

位置 小腿内侧,内踝尖上 2 寸,胫骨内侧缘后际凹陷中。

主治 月经不调,痛经,崩漏,阴挺,泄泻,便秘,睾丸肿痛。

Location：2 cun above the tip of the external malleolus, in the depression posterior to the medial border of tibia.

Indications: irregular menstruation, dysmenorrhea, uterin bleeding, prolapse of uterus, diarrhea, constipation, pain and swelling of testis.

KI9 筑宾 ZhùBīn(阴维脉郄穴)

位置 小腿内侧,太溪(KI3)直上 5 寸,比目鱼肌与跟腱之间。

主治 癫狂,足胫痛,疝痛。

Location: 5 cun directly above TàiXī (KI 3), between the musculus soleus and the tendo calcaneus.

Indications: mental disorder, pain in the foot and leg, pain due to hernia.

KI10 阴谷 YīnGǔ(合穴)

位置 膝后区,腘横纹上,半腱肌肌腱外侧缘。

主治 阳痿,疝痛,崩漏,小便不利。

Location: in the transverse crease of the popliteal fossa, at the lateral border of the tendon of m. semitendinosus.

Indications: impotence, pain due to hernia, uteri bleeding, urination disturbance.

K I

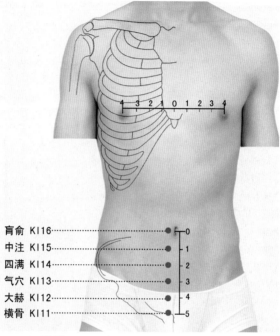

肓俞 KI16

中注 KI15

四满 KI14

气穴 KI13

大赫 KI12

横骨 KI11

KI11 横骨 HéngGǔ

位置 下腹部,脐中下 5 寸,前正中线旁开 0.5 寸。

主治 少腹满痛,小便不利,遗尿,遗精,阳痿,阴部痛。

Location：in the lower abdomen，5 cun below the umbilicus，0.5 cun lateral to the anterior midline.

Indications：distending pain of the lower abdomen，urination disturbance，enuresis，nocturnal emission，impotence，pain in the external genitalia.

KI12 大赫 DàHè

位置 下腹部,脐中下 4 寸,前正中线旁开 0.5 寸。

主治 遗精,阳痿,带下,阴部痛,阴挺。

Location：4 cun below the umbilicus，0.5 cun lateral to the anterior midline.

Indications: nocturnal emission, impotence, morbid leukorrhea, pain in the external genitalia, prolapse of uterus.

KI13 气穴 QìXué

位置　下腹部,脐中下 3 寸,前正中线旁开 0.5 寸。

主治　月经不调,痛经,小便不利,腹痛,泄泻。

Location: 3 cun below the umbilicus, 0.5 cun lateral to the anterior midline.

Indications: irregular menstruation, dysmenorrhea, urination disturbance, abdominal pain, diarrhea.

KI14 四满 SìMǎn

位置　下腹部,脐中下 2 寸,前正中线旁开 0.5 寸。

主治　腹痛,腹胀,泄泻,遗精,月经不调,痛经。

Location: 2 cun below the umbilicus, 0.5 cun lateral to the anterior midline.

Indications: abdominal pain or distension, diarrhea, nocturnal emission, irregular menstruation, dysmenorrhea.

KI15 中注 ZhōngZhù

位置　下腹部,脐中下 1 寸,前正中线旁开 0.5 寸。

主治　月经不调,腹痛,便秘。

Location: 1 cun below the umbilicus, 0.5 cun lateral to the anterior midline.

Indications: irregular menstruation, abdominal pain, constipation.

KI16 肓俞 HuāngShū

位置　腹部,脐中旁开 0.5 寸。

主治　腹痛,腹胀,呕吐,便秘,泄泻。

Location: 0.5 cun lateral to the umbilicus.

Indications: abdominal pain or distension, vomiting, constipation, diarrhea.

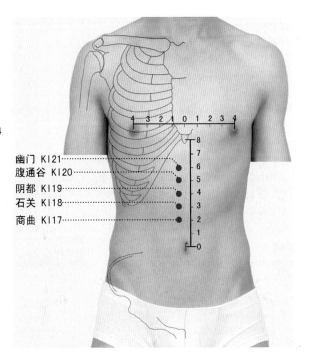

幽门 KI21
腹通谷 KI20
阴都 KI19
石关 KI18
商曲 KI17

KI17 商曲 ShāngQū

位置 上腹部,脐中上 2 寸,前正中线旁开 0.5 寸。

主治 腹痛,泄泻,便秘。

Location: in the upper abdomen, 2 cun above the umbilicus, 0.5 cun lateral to the anterior midline.

Indications: abdominal pain, diarrhea, constipation.

KI18 石关 ShíGuān

位置 上腹部,脐中上 3 寸,前正中线旁开 0.5 寸。

主治 呕吐,腹痛,便秘,产后腹痛,不孕。

Location: 3 cun above the umbilicus, 0.5 cun lateral to the anterior midline.

Indications: vomiting, abdominal pain, constipation, postpartum abdominal pain, sterility.

KI19 阴都 YīnDū

位置 上腹部,脐中上 4 寸,前正中线旁开 0.5 寸。

主治 肠鸣,腹痛,胃脘痛,便秘,呕吐。

Location: 4 cun above the umbilicus, 0.5 cun lateral to the anterior midline.

Indications: Borborygmus, abdominal pain, epigastric pain, constipation, vomiting.

KI20 腹通谷 FùTōnggǔ

位置 上腹部,脐中上 5 寸,前正中线旁开 0.5 寸。

主治 腹痛,腹胀,呕吐,消化不良。

Location: 5 cun above the umbilicus, 0.5 cun lateral to the anterior midline.

Indications: abdominal pain or distension, vomiting, indigestion.

KI21 幽门 YōuMén

位置 上腹部,脐中上 6 寸,前正中线旁开 0.5 寸。

主治 腹痛,腹胀,消化不良,呕吐,泄泻。

Location: 6 cun above the umbilicus, 0.5 cun lateral to the anterior midline.

Indications: abdominal pain or distension, indigestion, vomiting, diarrhea.

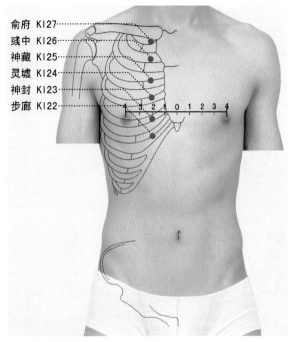

俞府 KI27
彧中 KI26
神藏 KI25
灵墟 KI24
神封 KI23
步廊 KI22

KI22 步廊 BùLáng

位置　胸部,第5肋间隙,前正中线旁开2寸。

主治　咳嗽,气喘,胸胁胀满。

Location: in the chest, in the fifth intercostal space, 2 cun lateral to the anterior midline.

Indications: cough, asthma, fullness in the chest and hypochondriac region.

KI23 神封 ShénFēng

位置　胸部,第4肋间隙,前正中线旁开2寸。

主治　咳嗽,气喘,胸胁胀满,乳痈。

Location: in the fourth intercostal space, 2 cun lateral to the anterior midline.

Indications: cough, asthma, fullness in the chest and hypochondriac region, mastitis.

KI24 灵墟 LíngXū

位置　胸部,第 3 肋间隙,前正中线旁开 2 寸。

主治　咳嗽,气喘,胸胁胀痛,乳痈。

Location: in the third intercostal space, 2 cun lateral to the anterior midline.

Indications: cough, asthma, fullness in the chest and hypochondriac region, mastitis.

KI25 神藏 ShénCáng

位置　胸部,第 2 肋间隙,前正中线旁开 2 寸。

主治　咳嗽,气喘,胸痛。

Location: In the second intercostal space, 2 cun lateral to the anterior midline.

Indications: cough, asthma, chest pain.

KI26 彧中 YùZhōng

位置　胸部,第 1 肋间隙,前正中线旁开 2 寸。

主治　咳嗽,气喘,痰壅,胸胁胀满。

Location: in the first intercostal space, 2 cun lateral to the anterior midline.

Indications: cough, asthma, accumulation of phlegm, fullness in the chest and hypochondriac region.

KI27 俞府 ShūFǔ

位置　胸部,锁骨下缘,前正中线旁开 2 寸。

主治　咳嗽,气喘,胸痛。

Location: in the depression at the lower border of the clavicle, 2 cun lateral to the anterior midline.

Indications: cough, asthma, pain in the chest.

KI

第 2 章　十四经腧穴 ·

Chapter II Acupoints of 14 Meridians

9. 手厥阴心包经 Pericardium Meridian of Hand Jueyin

手厥阴心包经分寸歌

心包穴起天池间,乳后旁一腋下三。
天泉曲腋下二寸,曲泽肘内横纹上。
郄门去腕方五寸,间使腕后四寸安。
内关去腕只二寸,大陵掌后两筋间。
劳宫屈中名指取,中冲中指之末端。

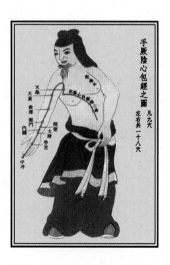

手厥阴心包经之图

凡九穴

左右共 一十八穴

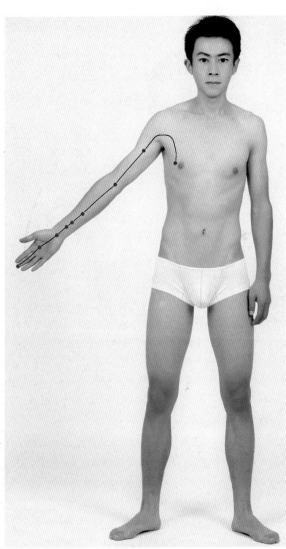

手厥阴心包经

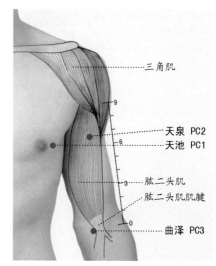

三角肌

天泉 PC2
天池 PC1

肱二头肌
肱二头肌肌腱

曲泽 PC3

PC1 天池 TiānChí

位置 胸部,第4肋间隙,前正中线旁开5寸。

主治 胸闷,胁痛,腋下肿痛。

Location：in the chest, in the fourth intercostal space, 5 cun lateral to the anterior midline.

Indications：oppressing feeling in the chest, pain in the hypochondriac region, swelling and pain of the axillary region.

PC2 天泉 TiānQuán

位置 臂前区,腋前纹头下2寸,肱二头肌的长、短头之间。

主治 心痛,胁胀,咳嗽,胸壁及上臂内侧痛。

Location：2 cun below the end of the anterior axillary fold, between the two heads of m. biceps brachii.

Indications：cardiac pain, distension in the hypochondriac region, cough, pain in the chest or the medial aspect of the arm.

PC

PC3 曲泽 QūZé(合穴)

位置 肘前区,肘横纹上,肱二头肌腱的尺侧缘凹陷中。

主治 心痛,心悸,热病,烦躁,胃痛,呕吐,肘臂疼痛,手臂震颤。

Location:in the anterior aspect of the elbow, in the transverse cubital crease, at the ulnar side of the tendon of m. biceps brachii.

Indications:cardiac pain, palpitation, febrile diseases, irritability, gastric pain, vomiting, pain in the elbow and arm, tremor of the hand and arm.

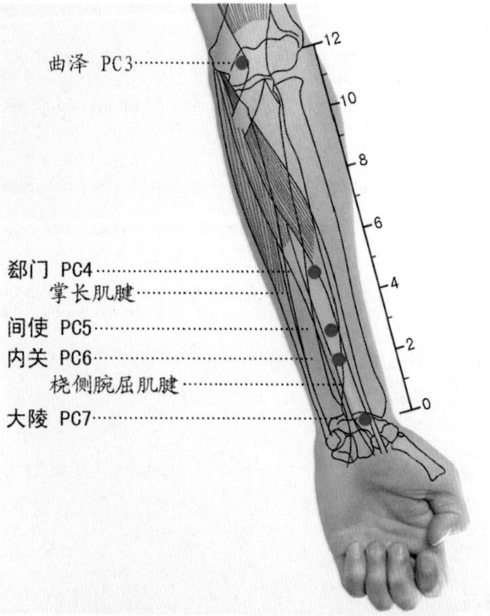

曲泽 PC3

郄门 PC4
掌长肌腱

间使 PC5

内关 PC6
桡侧腕屈肌腱

大陵 PC7

PC4 郄门 XìMén(郄穴)

位置 前臂前区,腕掌侧远端横纹上 5 寸,掌长肌腱与桡侧腕屈肌腱之间。

主治 心痛,心悸,衄血,呕血,咳血,胸痛,疔疮,癫证。

Location: 5 cun above the distal transverse crease of the wrist, between the tendons of m. palmaris longus and m. flexor carpi radialis.

Indications: cardiac pain, palpitation, epistaxis, hematemesis, haemoptysis, pain in the chest, furuncle, epilepsy.

PC5 间使 JiānShǐ(经穴)

位置 前臂前区,腕掌侧远端横纹上 3 寸,掌长肌腱与桡侧腕屈肌腱之间。

主治 心痛,心悸,胃痛,呕吐,热病,烦躁,疟疾,癫狂,腋肿,肘臂挛痛。

Location: 3 cun above the distal transverse crease of the wrist, between the tendons of m. palmaris longus and m. flexor carpi radialis.

Indications：cardiac pain, palpitation, gastric pain, vomiting, febrile diseases, irritability, malaria, mental disorder, swelling of the axilla, spasm of the elbow and arm.

PC6 内关 NèiGuān(络穴、八脉交会穴)

位置 前臂前区, 腕掌侧远端横纹上 2 寸, 掌长肌腱与桡侧腕屈肌腱之间。

主治 心痛, 心悸, 胸闷, 胃痛, 恶心, 呕吐, 呃逆, 热病, 烦躁, 疟疾。

Location：2 cun above the distal transverse crease of the wrist, between the tendons of m. palmaris longus and m. flexor radialis.

Indications：cardiac pain, palpitation, oppressing feeling in the chest, gastric pain, nausea, vomiting, hiccup, febrile diseases, irritability, malaria.

PC7 大陵 DàLíng(输穴、原穴)

位置 腕前区, 腕掌侧远端横纹上, 掌长肌腱与桡侧腕屈肌腱之间。

主治 心痛, 心悸, 胃痛, 呕吐, 痫证, 胸闷, 失眠, 烦躁, 口臭。

Location：at the distal transverse crease of the wrist, between the tendons of m. palmaris longus and m. flexor carpi radialis.

Indications：cardiac pain, palpitation, gastric pain, vomiting, epilepsy, oppressing feeling in the chest, insomnia, irritability, foul breath.

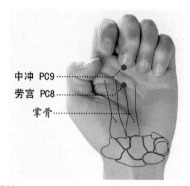

中冲 PC9
劳宫 PC8
掌骨

PC8 劳宫 LáoGōng（荥穴）

位置　掌区，横平第 3 掌指关节近端，第 2、3 掌骨之间偏于第 3 掌骨。

主治　心痛，癫狂，痫证，口疮，口臭，鹅掌风，呕吐。

Location：at the level of the proximal end of the third meta-carpophalangeal joint, between the 2nd and 3rd metacarpal bones but close to the latter.

Indications：cardiac pain, mental disorder, epilepsy, aphtha foul breath, tinea unguium, vomiting.

PC9 中冲 ZhōngChōng（井穴）

位置　手指，中指末端最高点。

主治　心痛，心烦，昏厥，舌强肿痛，热病，中暑，惊厥，掌中热。

Location：at the centre in the tip of the middle finger.

Indications：cardiac pain, irritability, loss of consciousness, stiffness and swelling of the tongue, febrile diseases, heat stroke, convulsion, feverish sensation in the palm.

PC

10. 手少阳三焦经 Triple Energizer Meridian of Hand Shaoyang

手少阳三焦经分寸歌

无名指外端关冲，液门小次指陷中。
中渚液门上一寸，阳池腕表陷中从。
外关腕后二寸取，腕后三寸支沟容。
支沟横外取会宗，空中一寸用心攻。
腕后四寸三阳络，四渎肘前五寸着。
天井肘外大骨后，骨罅中间一寸摸。
肘后二寸清冷渊，肘后五寸是消泺。
臑会肩前三寸量，肩髎臑上陷中央。
耳门耳缺前起肉，和髎耳前锐发乡。
欲知丝竹空何在，眉梢陷中不须量。

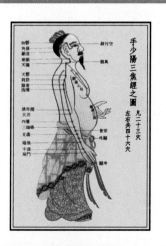

手少陽三焦經之圖
凡二十三穴
左右共四十六穴

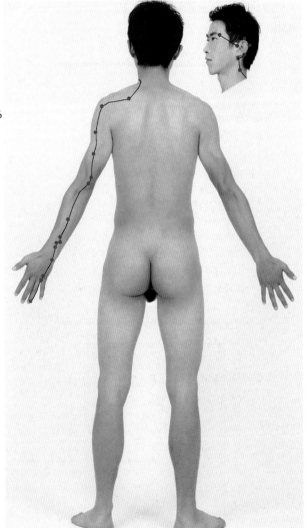

TE

手少阳三焦经

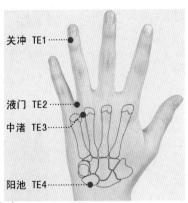

关冲 TE1

液门 TE2

中渚 TE3

阳池 TE4

TE1 关冲 GuānChōng(井穴)

位置 手指,第4指末节尺侧,指甲根角侧上方0.1寸(指寸)。

主治 头痛,目赤,咽喉肿痛,舌强,热病,心烦。

Location：at the ulnar side of the terminal phalanx of the ring finger，0.1 cun from the corner of nail.

Indications：headache, red eyes, sore throat, stiffness of the tongue, febrile diseases, irritability.

TE2 液门 YèMén(荥穴)

位置 手背,第4、5指间,指蹼缘上方赤白肉际凹陷中。

主治 头痛、目赤,暴聋、咽喉肿痛,疟疾,手臂痛。

Location：in the depression distal to the web margin between the ring and little fingers, at the junction of the red and white skin.

Indications：headache, redness of the eyes, sudden deafness, sore throat, malaria, pain in the arm.

TE3 中渚 ZhōngZhǔ(输穴)

位置 手背,第4、5掌骨间,第4掌指关节近端凹陷中。

主治 头痛,目赤,耳聋,耳鸣,咽喉肿痛,热病,肘臂痛,手指不能屈伸。

Location：in the dorsum of hand between the fourth and fifth metacarpal bones, in the depression proximal to the fourth metacarpophalangeal joint.

Indications：headache, redness of the eyes, deafness, tinnitus, sore throat, febrile diseases, pain in the elbow and arm, motor impairment of fingers.

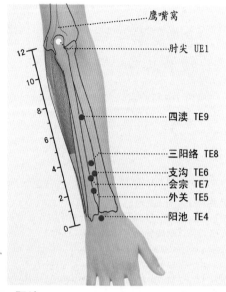

鹰嘴窝

肘尖 UE1

四渎 TE9

三阳络 TE8

支沟 TE6

会宗 TE7

外关 TE5

阳池 TE4

TE4 阳池 YángChí(原穴)

位置 腕后区,腕背侧远端横纹上,指伸肌腱的尺侧缘凹陷中。

主治 肩臂痛,腕痛,疟疾,耳聋,消渴。

Location: in the distal dorsal crease of the wrist, in the depression lateral to the tendon of m. extensor digitorum communis.

Indications: pain in the arm, shoulder or wrist, malaria, deafness, diabetes.

TE5 外关 WàiGuān(络穴,八脉交会穴)

位置 前臂后区,腕背侧远端横纹上2寸,尺骨与桡骨间隙中点。

主治 热病,头痛,颊痛,落枕,耳鸣,胁肋痛,肘臂屈伸不利,手指疼痛。

Location: 2 cun proximal to the dorsal crease of the wrist, between the radius and ulna.

Indications: febrile diseases, headache, pain in the cheek, stiff neck, tinnitus, pain in the hypochondriac region, motor impairment of the elbow and arm, pain of the fingers.

TE6 支沟 ZhīGōu(经穴)

位置　前臂后区,腕背侧远端横纹上 3 寸,尺骨与桡骨间隙中点。

主治　耳鸣,耳聋,胁肋痛,呕吐,便秘,热病,暴暗。

Location：3 cun proximal to the dorsal crease of the wrist, between the radius and ulna.

Indications：tinnitus, deafness, pain in the hypochondriac region, vomiting, constipation, febrile diseases, sudden loss of voice.

TE7 会宗 HuìZōng(郄穴)

位置　前臂后区,腕背侧远端横纹上 3 寸,尺骨桡侧缘。

主治　耳聋,耳痛,臂痛。

Location：3 cun proximal to the dorsal crease of the wrist, at the radial border of the ulna.

Indications：deafness, ear pain, pain of the arm.

TE8 三阳络 SānYángLuò

位置　前臂背侧,腕背横纹上 4 寸,尺骨与桡骨之间。

主治　耳聋,暴暗,胸胁痛,手臂痛,齿痛。

Location：4 cun proximal to the dorsal crease of the wrist, between the radius and ulna.

Indications：deafness, sudden loss of voice, pain in the chest and hypochondriac regions, pain in the arm, toothache.

TE9 四渎 SìDú

位置　前臂后区,肘尖(EX‐UX1)下 5 寸,尺骨与桡骨间隙中点。

主治　耳聋,齿痛,偏头痛,暴暗,前臂痛。

Location：5 cun distal to ZhǒuJiān (EX‐UX1), between the radius and ulna.

Indications：deafness, toothache, migraine, sudden loss of voice, pain in the forearm.

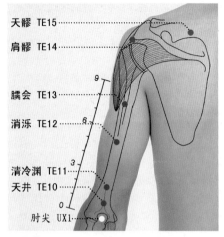

天髎 TE15

肩髎 TE14

臑会 TE13

消泺 TE12

清冷渊 TE11

天井 TE10

肘尖 UX1

TE10 天井 TiānJǐng(合穴)

位置 肘后区,肘尖(EX – UX1)上1寸凹陷中。

主治 偏头痛,颈项、肩臂痛,痫证,瘰疬,气瘿。

Location：in the depression 1 cun proximal to ZhǒuJiān (EX – UX1).

Indications：migraine, pain in the neck, shoulder or arm, epilepsy, scrofula, goiter.

TE11 清冷渊 QīngLěngYuān

位置 臂后区,肘尖(EX – UX1)与肩峰角连线上,肘尖(EX – UX1)直上2寸。

主治 肩臂痛不举,偏头痛。

Location：in the line connecting ZhǒuJiān (EX – UX1) and the acromial angle, 2 cun directly proximal to ZhǒuJiān (EX – UX1).

Indications：motor impairment and pain of the shoulder and arm, migraine.

TE12 消泺 XiāoLuò

位置 臂后区,肘尖(EX – UX1)与肩峰角连线上,肘尖(EX – UX1)直上5寸。

TE

主治 头痛、颈项强痛,臂痛不举。

Location: in the line connecting ZhǒuJiān（EX - UX1）and the acromial angle, 5 cun directly proximal to ZhǒuJiān（EX - UX1）.

Indications: headache, stiffness and pain of the neck, motor impairment and pain of the shoulder and arm.

TE13 臑会 NàoHuì

位置 臂后区,肩峰角下 3 寸,三角肌的后下缘。

主治 气瘿,肩臂疼痛。

Location: 3 cun distal to the acromial angle, at the posteroinferior border of m. deltoideus.

Indications: goiter, pain in the shoulder and arm.

TE14 肩髎 JiānLiáo

位置 三角肌区,肩峰角与肱骨大结节两骨间凹陷中。

主治 肩臂疼痛不举,上肢痿痹。

Location:in the deltoid muscle, in the depression between the acromial angle and the greater tubercle of the humerus.

Indications: pain, motor impairment of the shoulder and upper limbs.

TE15 天髎 TiānLiáo

位置 肩胛区,肩胛骨上角骨际凹陷中。

主治 肩肘痛,颈项强痛。

Location: in the depression at the superior angle of the scapula.

Indications: pain in the shoulder and elbow, stiffness and pain of the neck.

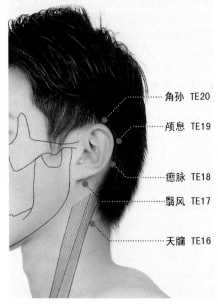

角孙 TE20

颅息 TE19

瘛脉 TE18

翳风 TE17

天牖 TE16

TE16 天牖 TiānYǒu

位置 颈部,横平下颌角,胸锁乳突肌的后缘凹陷中。

主治 头痛,项强,面肿,目昏,暴聋。

Location: in the lateral side of the neck, at the level of the mandibular angle, in the depression at the posterior border of sternocleidomastoid muscle.

Indications: headache, neck rigidity, facial swelling, blurred vision, sudden deafness.

TE17 翳风 YìFēng

位置 颈部,耳垂后方,乳突下端前方凹陷中。

主治 耳鸣,耳聋,口眼歪斜,齿痛,颊肿,瘰疬,牙关不利。

Location: posterior to the lobule of the ear, in the depression anterior to the lower end of the mastoid process.

Indications: tinnitus, deafness, facial paralysis, toothache, swelling of the cheek, scrofula, trismus.

TE18 瘈脉 ChìMài

位置 头部，乳突中央，角孙(TE20)至翳风(TE17)延耳轮弧形连线上 2/3 与下 1/3 的交点处。

主治 头痛，耳鸣，耳聋，小儿惊痫。

Location: in the center of the mastoid process, at the junction of the upper two-thirds and lower one-third of the curve formed by JiǎoSūn(TE20)and YìFēng(TE17)behind the helix.

Indications: headache, tinnitus, deafness, infantile convulsion.

TE19 颅息 LúXī

位置 头部，角孙(TE20)至翳风(TE17)延耳轮弧形连线上 1/3 与下 2/3 的交点处。

主治 头痛，耳鸣，耳聋，耳痛，小儿惊痫。

Location: in the head, at the junction of the upper one-third and lower two-thirds of the curve formed by JiǎoSūn(TE20) and YìFēng(TE17)behind the helix.

Indications: headache, tinnitus, deafness, ear pain, infantile convulsion.

TE20 角孙 JiǎoSūn

位置 头部，耳尖正对发际处。

主治 耳鸣，目赤肿痛，龈肿，齿痛，疟腮。

Location: directly above the ear apex, within the hairline.

Indications: tinnitus, redness, pain and swelling of the eye, swelling of gum, toothache, parotitis.

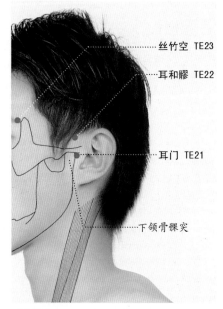

丝竹空 TE23

耳和髎 TE22

耳门 TE21

下颌骨髁突

TE21 耳门 ĚrMén

位置 耳区,耳屏上切迹与下颌骨髁突之间的凹陷中。

主治 耳鸣,耳聋,齿痛。

Location: in the depression between the supratragic notch and the condyloid process of the mandible.

Indications: tinnitus, deafness, toothache.

TE22 耳和髎 ĚrHéLiáo

位置 头部,鬓发后缘,耳廓根的前方,颞浅动脉的后缘。

主治 偏头痛,耳鸣,牙关拘急。

Location: at the posterior border of the hairline of the temple where the superficial temporal artery passes, anterior to the root of the auricle.

Indications: migraine, tinnitus, trismus.

TE23 丝竹空 SīZhúKōng

位置　面部,眉梢凹陷中。

主治　头痛,目赤痛,目眩,齿痛,口眼歪斜。

Location：in the depression at the lateral end of the eyebrow.

Indications：headache, redness and pain of the eye, blurred vision, toothache, facial paralysis.

11. 足少阳胆经 Gallbladder Meridian of Foot Shaoyang

足少阳胆经分寸歌

外眦五分瞳子髎，耳前陷中听会绕。

上关上行一寸明，内斜曲角颔厌绕。

斜后下行悬颅定，悬厘颅下半寸徽。

曲鬓耳前发际上，入发寸半率骨邈。

天冲率后斜五分，浮白率下一寸瞧。

枕骨之上头窍阴，完骨耳后发际认。

入发四分须记真，本神神庭旁三寸。

和发五分眦上凭，阳白眉上一寸论。

却与瞳子直相对，入发五分头临泣。

旁开相对到神庭，临后一寸目窗位。

窗后一寸正营穴，正营之后承灵逢。

相去寸半见甲乙，风池直上寻脑空。

夹脑户旁二寸间，风池上尖角陷。

肩井肩上陷解中，大骨之前寸半辨。

渊腋腋下三寸从，再从渊腋横前测。

相隔一寸辄筋逢，日月期门下一肋。

十二肋端是京门，章下寸八寻带脉。

带下三寸五枢真，维道章下五三择。

章下八三居髎名，环跳髀枢宛中陷。

风市垂手中指寻，中渎膝上五寸鉴。

阳关阳陵上三寸，阳陵膝下一寸量。

腓骨头前陷中取，阳交踝上七寸乡。

此系斜属三阳络，外丘踝上七寸长。

踝上五寸光明着，踝上四寸阳辅当。

踝上三寸悬钟列，丘墟踝下陷中商。

丘下三寸足临泣，侠溪之上寸五藏。

临下五分地五会，会下一寸侠溪疆。

足窍阴穴在何处，小次趾外侧角量。

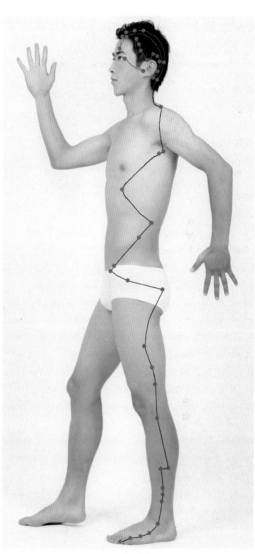

足少阳胆经

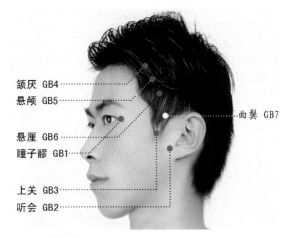

颔厌 GB4

悬颅 GB5

曲鬓 GB7

悬厘 GB6

瞳子髎 GB1

上关 GB3

听会 GB2

GB1 瞳子髎 TóngZiLiáo

位置 面部,目外眦外侧 0.5 寸凹陷中。

主治 头痛,目赤痛,迎风流泪,视力衰退,口眼歪斜。

Location: in the depression 0.5 cun lateral to the outer canthus.

Indications: headache, redness and pain of the eye, failing of vision, lacrimation induced by wind, facial paralysis.

GB2 听会 TīngHuì

位置 面部,耳屏间切迹与下颌骨髁突之间的凹陷中。

主治 耳聋,耳鸣,齿痛,牙关不利,痄腮,口眼歪斜。

Location: in the face, in the depression between the intertragic notch and the condyloid process of the mandible.

Indications: deafness, tinnitus, toothache, motor impairment of the temporomandibular joint, parotitis, facial paralysis.

GB3 上关 ShàngGuān

位置 面部,颧弓的上缘中央凹陷中。

主治 头痛,耳聋,耳鸣,口眼歪斜,齿痛。

Location: in the depression at the midpoint of the upper border of the zygomatic arch.

Indications: headache, deafness, tinnitus, facial paralysis,

GB

toothache.

GB4 颔厌 HànYàn

位置 头部,从头维(ST8)至曲鬓(GB7)的弧形连线(其弧度与鬓发弧度相应)的上 1/4 与下 3/4 的交点处。

主治 偏头痛,目眩,耳鸣,目外眦痛,齿痛,痫证。

Location: at the junction of the upper one-fourth and lower three-fourths of the curve formed by TóuWéi (ST8) and QǔBìn (GB7).

Indications: migraine, vertigo, tinnitus, pain in the outer canthus, toothache, epilepsy.

GB5 悬颅 XuánLú

位置 头部,从头维(ST8)至曲鬓(GB7)的弧形连线(其弧度与鬓发弧度相应)的中点处。

主治 偏头痛,目外眦痛,面肿。

Location: midpoint of the curve formed by TóuWéi (ST8) and QǔBìn (GB7).

Indications: migraine, pain in the outer canthus, facial swelling.

GB6 悬厘 XuánLí

位置 头部,从头维(ST8)至曲鬓(GB7)的弧形连线(其弧度与鬓发弧度相应)的上 3/4 与下 1/4 的交点处。

主治 偏头痛,目外眦痛,耳鸣,善嚏。

Location: at the junction of the upper three-fourths and lower one-fourth of the curve formed by TóuWéi (ST8) and QǔBìn (GB7).

Indications: migraine, pain in the outer canthus, tinnitus, frequent sneezing.

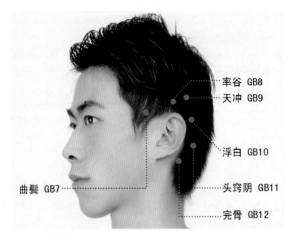

率谷 GB8
天冲 GB9
浮白 GB10
头窍阴 GB11
完骨 GB12
曲鬓 GB7

GB7 曲鬓 QǔBìn

位置 头部,耳前鬓角发际后缘与耳尖水平线的交点处。

主治 头痛,颊颔肿,牙关紧闭,小儿惊风。

Location：in the head, at a crossing point of the posterior border of the hairline anterior to the ear and the horizontal line along the ear apex.

Indications：headache, swelling of the cheek, trismus, infantile convulsion.

GB8 率谷 ShuàiGǔ

位置 头部,耳尖直上入发际1.5寸。

主治 偏头痛,眩晕,呕吐,小儿惊风。

Location：in the head, superior to the ear apex, 1.5 cun within the hairline.

Indications：migraine, dizziness, vertigo, vomiting, infantile convulsion.

GB9 天冲 TiānChōng

位置 头部,耳根后缘直上,入发际2寸。

主治 头痛,痫证,齿龈肿痛。

Location：in the head, directly above the posterior border of the auricle, 2 cun within the hairline.

Indications：headache, epilepsy, swelling and pain of the gums.

GB10 浮白 FúBái

位置 头部，耳后乳突的后上方，从天冲(GB9)至完骨(GB12)的弧形连线(其弧度与耳郭弧度相应)的上 1/3 与下 2/3 交点处。

主治 头痛，耳鸣，耳聋。

Location：posterosuperior to the mastoid process, at the junction of the upper one-third and lower two-thirds of the curve formed by TiānChōng(GB9) and WánGǔ(GB12).

Indications：headache, tinnitus, deafness.

GB11 头窍阴 TóuQiàoYīn

位置 头部，耳后乳突的后上方，从天冲(GB9)至完骨(GB12)的弧形连线(其弧度与耳郭弧度相应)的上 2/3 与下 1/3 交点处。

主治 头项痛，耳鸣，耳聋，耳痛。

Location：posterosuperior to the mastoid process, at the junction of the upper two-thirds and lower one-third of the curve formed by TiānChōng(GB9) and WánGǔ(GB12).

Indications：pain of the head and neck, tinnitus, deafness, ear pain.

GB12 完骨 WánGǔ

位置 头部，耳后乳突的后下方凹陷中。

主治 头痛，失眠，颊肿，耳后痛，口眼歪斜，齿痛。

Location：in the depression posteroinferior to the mastoid process.

Indications：headache, insomnia, swelling of the cheek, retro-auricular pain, facial paralysis, toothache.

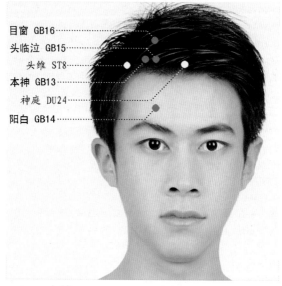

目窗 GB16
头临泣 GB15
头维 ST8
本神 GB13
神庭 DU24
阳白 GB14

GB13 本神 BěnShén

位置 头部,前发际上0.5寸,头正中线旁开3寸。

主治 头痛,失眠,目眩,痫证。

Location：0.5 cun within the hairline of the forehead, 3 cun lateral to the anterior hairline.

Indications：headache, insomnia, vertigo, epilepsy.

GB14 阳白 YángBái

位置 头部,眉上1寸,瞳孔直上。

主治 前额痛,眉棱骨痛,目痛,目眩,眼睑下垂,迎风流泪。

Location：in the forehead, 1 cun directly above the midpoint of the eyebrow, directly above the pupil.

Indications：pain in the forehead, pain in the supraorbital ridge, eye pain, vertigo, ptosis of the eyelids, lacrimation induced by wind.

GB15 头临泣 TóuLínQì

位置　头部,前发际上 0.5 寸,瞳孔直上。

主治　头痛,目眩,迎风流泪,目外眦痛,鼻塞,鼻渊。

Location: 0.5 cun above the anterior hairline, directly above the pupil.

Indications: headache, vertigo, lacrimation induced by wind, pain in the outer canthus, nasal obstruction, rhinorrhea.

GB16 目窗 MùChuāng

位置　头部,前发际上 1.5 寸,瞳孔直上。

主治　头痛,眩晕,目赤痛,鼻塞。

Location: 1.5 cun above the anterior hairline, directly above the pupil.

Indications: headache, dizziness, vertigo, redness and pain of the eye, nasal obstruction.

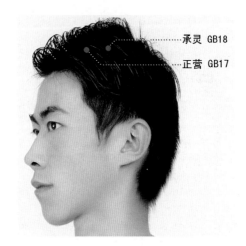

承灵 GB18

正营 GB17

GB17 正营 ZhèngYíng

位置 头部，前发际上 2.5 寸，瞳孔直上。

主治 偏头痛，眩晕。

Location：2.5 cun above the anterior hairline, directly above the pupil.

Indications：migraine, dizziness, vertigo.

GB18 承灵 ChéngLíng

位置 头部，前发际上 4 寸，瞳孔直上。

主治 头痛，眩晕，鼻衄，鼻渊。

Location：4 cun above the anterior hairline, directly above the pupil.

Indications：headache, dizziness, vertigo, epistaxis, rhinorrhea.

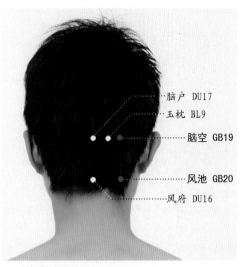

脑户 DU17
玉枕 BL9
脑空 GB19
风池 GB20
风府 DU16

GB19 脑空 NǎoKōng

位置 头部,横平枕外隆凸的上缘,风池(GB20)直上。

主治 头痛,项强,眩晕,目痛,耳鸣,痫证。

Location: at the level of the upper border of external occipital protuberance, directly above FēngChí(GB20).

Indications: headache, neck rigidity, dizziness, vertigo, eye pain, tinnitus, epilepsy.

GB20 风池 FēngChí

位置 项后区,枕骨之下,胸锁乳突肌与斜方肌上端之间的凹陷中。

主治 头痛,眩晕,失眠,目视不明,目赤痛。

Location: inferior to the occipital bone, in the depression between the upper portion of m. sternocleidomastoideus and m. trapezius.

Indications: headache, dizziness, vertigo, insomnia, blurred vision, redness and pain of the eye.

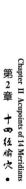

GB

第2章 十四经腧穴 ·

Chapter II Acupoints of 14 Meridians

145

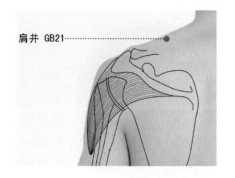

肩井 GB21

GB21 肩井 JiānJǐng

位置　肩胛区，第 7 颈椎棘突与肩峰最外侧点连线的中点。

主治　颈项强痛，肩背痛，乳痈，中风。

Location：in the shoulder，at the midpoint of the line connecting the spinous process of the seventh thoracic verte-bra and the ac-romion.

Indications：pain and rigidity of the neck，pain in the shoulder and back，mastitis，stroke.

GB

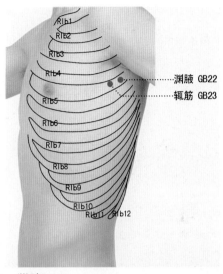

GB22 渊腋 YuānYè

位置　胸外侧区,第 4 肋间隙中,在腋中线上。

主治　胸满,腋下肿,胁痛,臂痛不举。

Location：in the 4th intercostal space, at the mid-axillary line.

Indications：fullness in the chest, swelling of the axillary region, pain in the hypochondriac region, pain and motor impairment of the arm.

GB23 辄筋 ZhéJīn

位置　胸外侧区,第 4 肋间隙中,腋中线前 1 寸。

主治　胸满,胁痛,气喘。

Location：in the 4th intercostal space, 1 cun anterior to the mid-axillary line.

Indications：fullness in the chest, pain in the hypochondriac region, asthma.

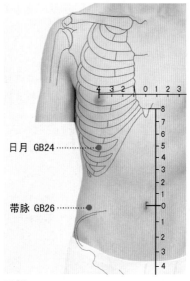

日月 GB24

带脉 GB26

GB24 日月 RìYuè(胆募穴)

位置 胸部,第 7 肋间隙中,前正中线旁开 4 寸。

主治 胁痛,呕吐,吞酸,呕逆,黄疸,乳痛。

Location：in the seventh intercostal space, 4 cun lateral to the anterior midline.

Indications：pain in the hypochondriac region, vomiting, acid regurgitation, hiccup, jaundice, mastitis.

GB25 京门 JīngMén(肾募穴)

位置 上腹部,第 12 肋骨游离端的下际。

主治 腹胀,肠鸣,泄泻,腰胁痛。

Location：in the upper abdomen, inferior to the free end of the twelfth rib.

Indications：abdominal distension, borborygmus, diarrhea, pain in the lumbar and hypochondriac region.

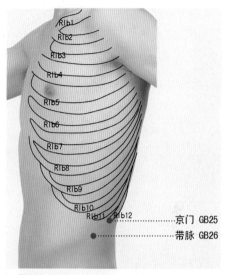

RIb1
RIb2
RIb3
RIb4
RIb5
RIb6
RIb7
RIb8
RIb9
RIb10
RIb11 RIb12 .... 京门 GB25
.... 带脉 GB26

GB26 带脉 DàiMài

位置　侧腹部,第 11 肋骨游离端垂线与脐水平线的交点上。

主治　月经不调,闭经,赤白带下,腹痛,疝气,腰胁痛。

Location: at the crossing point of a vertical line through the free end of the eleventh rib and a horizontal line through the umbilicus.

Indications: irregular menstruation, amenorrhea, morbid leukorrhea, abdominal pain, hernia, pain in the lumbar and hypochondriac region.

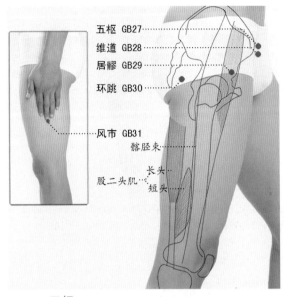

五枢 GB27
维道 GB28
居髎 GB29
环跳 GB30
风市 GB31
髂胫束
股二头肌 — 长头
短头

GB

GB27 五枢 WǔShū

位置 下腹部,横平脐下3寸,髂前上棘内侧。

主治 赤白带下,腰胯痛,少腹痛,疝气,便秘。

Location: in the lower abdomen, 3 cun below the umbilicus, at the medial side of the anterior superior lilac spine.

Indications: morbid leukorrhea, pain in the lumbar or hip, lower abdominal pain, hernia, constipation.

GB28 维道 WéiDào

位置 下腹部,髂前上棘内下0.5寸。

主治 带下,少腹痛,疝气,阴挺。

Location: in the lower abdomen, 0.5 cun medial and inferior to the anterior superior lilac spine.

Indications: morbid leukorrhea, lower abdominal pain, hernia, prolapse of uterus.

GB29 居髎 JūLiáo

位置　臀区,髂前上棘与股骨大转子最凸点连线的中点处。

主治　腰腿痹痛,瘫痪,下肢痿痹。

Location: in the depression of the midpoint between the anterior superior iliac spine and the prominence of the great trochanter.

Indications: pain in the lumbar or thigh, muscular atrophy or pain of the lower limbs.

GB30 环跳 HuánTiào

位置　臀区,股骨大转子最凸点与骶管裂孔连线的 1/3 与内 2/3 交点处。

主治　腰腿痛,下肢痿痹,半身不遂。

Location: at the junction of the lateral one-third and medial two-thirds of the line connecting the prominence of the great trochanter and the hiatus of the sacrum.

Indications: sciatica, muscular atrophy, pain or hemiplegia of the lower limbs.

GB31 风市 FēngShì

位置　股部,直立垂手,掌心贴于大腿时,中指尖所指凹陷中,髂胫束后缘。

主治　腰腿疼痛,下肢痿痹,皮肤瘙痒。

Location: in the thigh. When a patient is standing erect with the hands closed on the lateral aspect of the thigh, this point is where the tip of the middle finger touches and at the posterior border of the tractus iliotibialis.

Indications: pain in the thigh and lumbar region, paralysis or pain of the lower limbs,Itchy skin.

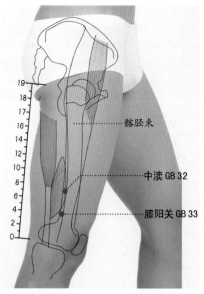

髂胫束

中渎 GB 32

膝阳关 GB 33

GB32 中渎 ZhōngDú

位置 股部,腘横纹上 7 寸,髂胫束后缘。

主治 腿膝疼痛,痿痹不仁,半身不遂。

Location: in the lateral aspect of the thigh, 7 cun above the transverse crease of the popliteal fossa, at the posterior border of the tractus iliotibialis.

Indications: pain of the thigh or knee, numbness and weakness of the lower limbs, hemiplegia.

GB33 膝阳关 XīYángGuān

位置 膝部,股骨外上髁后上缘,股二头肌腱与髂胫束之间的凹陷中。

主治 膝肿痛,小腿麻木。

Indications: in the knee, at the posterior border above the external epicondyle of femur, in the depression between the tendon of biceps femoris and the tractus iliotibialis.

Indications: swelling and pain of the knee, numbness of the leg.

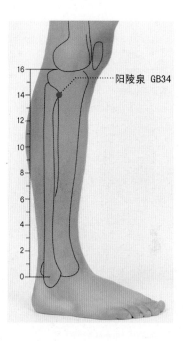

阳陵泉 GB34

GB34 阳陵泉 YángLíngQuán(合穴、筋会穴)

位置 小腿外侧,腓骨头前下方凹陷中。

主治 半身不遂,下肢痿痹、麻木,膝膑肿痛,胁肋痛,口苦,呕吐,黄疸,小儿惊风。

Location: in the lateral aspect of the leg, in the depression anterior and inferior to the head of the fibula.

Indications: hemiplegia, weakness, numbness and pain of the lower limbs, swelling and pain of the knee, hypochondriac pain, bitter taste in the mouth, vomiting, jaundice, infantile convulsion.

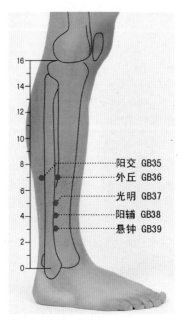

阳交 GB35
外丘 GB36
光明 GB37
阳辅 GB38
悬钟 GB39

GB35 阳交 YángJiāo(阳维脉郄穴)

位置 小腿外侧,外踝尖上7寸,腓骨后缘。

主治 胸胁胀满,下肢痿痹。

Location：7 cun above the tip of the external malleolus，at the posterior border of the fibula.

Indications：fullness in the chest and hypochondriac region，muscular atrophy，paralysis or pain of the lower limbs.

GB36 外丘 WàiQiū(郄穴)

位置 小腿外侧,外踝尖上7寸,腓骨前缘。

主治 胸胁痛,颈项痛,腿痛。

Location：7 cun above the tip of the external malleolus，at the anterior border of the fibula.

Indications：pain in the chest，hypochondriac region，neck or leg.

GB37 光明 GuāngMíng (络穴)

位置 小腿外侧，外踝尖上5寸，腓骨前缘。

主治 膝痛，下肢痿痹，目视不明，目痛，夜盲，乳房胀痛。

Location: 5 cun directly above the tip of the external malleolus, on the anterior border of the fibula.

Indications: knee pain, muscular atrophy, motor impairment or pain of the lower limbs, blurred vision, ophthalmalgia, night blindness, distending pain in the breast.

GB38 阳辅 YángFǔ (经穴)

位置 小腿外侧，外踝尖上4寸，腓骨前缘。

主治 偏头痛，目外眦痛，腋下痛，腰痛，胸胁及下肢外侧痛。

Location: 4 cun above the tip of the external malleolus, at the anterior border of the fibula.

Indications: migraine, pain in the outer canthus, the axillary region, chest, hypochondriac region, lumbar or the lower limbs.

GB39 悬钟 XuánZhōng (髓会穴)

位置 小腿外侧，外踝尖上3寸，腓骨前缘。

主治 中风，半身不遂，颈项痛，腹胀，胁痛，下肢痿痹，足胫挛痛，脚气。

Location: 3 cun above the tip of the external malleolus, at the anterior border of the fibula.

Indications: apoplexy, hemiplegia, neck pain, abdominal distension, pain in the hypochondriac region, muscular atrophy or pain in the lower limbs, spastic pain of the leg, beriberi.

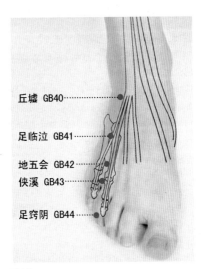

丘墟 GB40

足临泣 GB41

地五会 GB42

侠溪 GB43

足窍阴 GB44

GB40 丘墟 QiūXū(原穴)

位置 踝区,外踝的前下方,趾长伸肌腱的外侧凹陷中。

主治 颈项痛,腋下肿,胸胁痛,呕吐,嗳酸,外踝肿痛,疟疾。

Location: distal and inferior to the external malleolus, in the depression at the lateral side of the tendon of m. extensor digitorum longus.

Indications: neck pain, swelling in the axillary region, pain in the chest and hypochondriac region, vomiting, acid regurgitation, swelling and pain in the external malleolus, malaria.

GB41 足临泣 ZúLínQì(输穴、八脉交会穴)

位置 足背,第4、5跖骨底结合部的前方,第5趾长伸肌腱外侧凹陷中。

主治 头痛,目眩,目外眦痛,胁肋痛,乳房胀痛,月经不调,足趾挛痛。

Location: distal to the junction of the fourth and fifth metatarsal bones, in the depression lateral to the tendon of m. extensor digiti minimi of the foot.

Indications: headache, vertigo, pain in the outer canthus or hypochondriac region, distending pain in the breast, irregular menstruation, spastic pain of the foot and toe.

GB42 地五会 DìWǔHuì

位置 足背,第 4、5 跖骨间,第 4 跖趾关节近端凹陷中。

主治 目眦痛,耳鸣,乳房胀痛,足跗肿痛。

Location: between the fourth and fifth metatarsal bones, in the depression at the proximal fourth metatarsophalangeal joint.

Indications: pain in the canthus, tinnitus, distending pain in the breast, swelling and pain in the dorsum of foot.

GB43 侠溪 XiáXī (荥穴)

位置 足背,第 4、5 趾间,趾蹼缘后方赤白肉际处。

主治 头痛,眩晕,目外眦痛,耳鸣,耳聋,颊肿,胁肋痛,乳房胀痛,热病。

Location: proximal to the web margin between the fourth and fifth toes, at the junction of the red and white skin.

Indications: headache, dizziness, vertigo, pain in the outer canthus, tinnitus, deafness, swelling of the cheek, pain in the hypochondriac region, distending pain in the breast, febrile diseases.

GB44 足窍阴 ZúQiàoYīn(井穴)

位置 足背,第 4 趾末节外侧,趾甲根角侧后 0.1 寸(指寸)。

主治 偏头痛,耳聋,耳鸣,目痛,多梦,热病。

Location: at the lateral side of the terminal phalanx of fourth toe, 0.1 cun from the corner of nail.

Indications: migraine, deafness, tinnitus, ophthalmalgia, dream-disturbed sleep, febrile diseases.

12．足厥阴肝经 Liver Meridian of Foot Jueyin

足厥阴肝经分寸歌

足大指商大敦在，行间大趾缝中藏。
太冲本节后二寸，踝前一寸中封量。
蠡沟踝上五寸是，中都踝上七寸长。
膝关阴陵后一寸，曲泉屈膝横纹彰。
阴包膝上方四寸，气冲三寸五里裹。
阴廉冲下只二寸，急脉二寸半阴旁。
章门平脐肋端取，乳下两寸期门方。

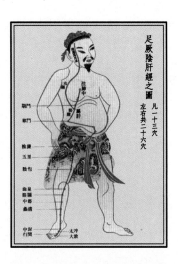

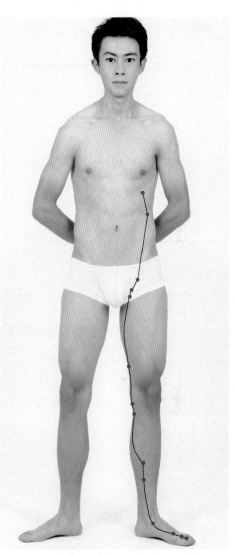

足厥阴肝经

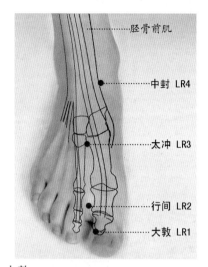

胫骨前肌

中封 LR4

太冲 LR3

行间 LR2

大敦 LR1

LR1 大敦 DàDūn(井穴)

位置 足趾,大趾末节外侧,趾甲根角侧后方 0.1 寸(指寸)。

主治 疝气,遗尿,崩漏,阴挺,痫证。

Location：at the lateral side of the terminal phalanx of the big toe, 0.1 cun from the corner of nail.

Indications：hernia, enuresis, uterine bleeding, prolapse of uterus, epilepsy.

LR2 行间 XíngJiān(荥穴)

位置 足背,第 1、2 趾间,趾蹼缘后方赤白肉际处。

主治 头痛,眩晕,胁痛,腹胀,疝痛,小便不利,月经不调,痫证,失眠。

Location：at the dorsum of foot, proximal to the web margin between the first and second toes, at the junction of the red and white skin.

Indications：headache, dizziness, vertigo, pain in the hypochondrium, abdominal distension, pain due to hernia, urination disturbance, irregular menstruation, epilepsy, insomnia.

LR

LR3 太冲 TàiChōng(输穴、原穴)

位置　足背侧,第1、2跖骨间,跖骨底结合部前方凹陷中,或触及动脉搏动。

主治　头痛,眩晕,失眠,目赤肿痛,胁痛,疝气,小便不利,痫证,内踝前缘痛。

Location：at the dorsum of foot, in the depression distal to the junction of the first and second metatarsal bones, where the artery passes.

Indications：headache, dizziness, vertigo, insomnia, redness, swelling and pain of the eye, pain in the hypochondriac region, hernia, urination disturbance, epilepsy, pain in the anterior aspect of the medial malleolus.

LR4 中封 ZhōngFēng(经穴)

位置　踝区,内踝前,胫骨前肌肌腱的内侧凹陷处。

主治　疝气,阴部痛,遗精,小便不利,胁肋胀痛。

Location：anterior to the medial malleolus, in the depression at the medial side of the tendon of m. tibialis anterior.

Indications：hernia, pain in the external genitalia, nocturnal emission, urination disturbance, distending pain in the hypochondrium.

LR

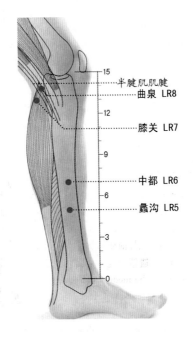

半腱肌肌腱
曲泉 LR8
膝关 LR7
中都 LR6
蠡沟 LR5

LR5 蠡沟 LíGōu（络穴）

位置　小腿内侧，内踝尖上 5 寸，胫骨内侧面的中央。

主治　小便不利，遗尿，疝气，月经不调，赤白带下，外阴瘙痒，足胫痿痹。

Location：5 cun above the tip of the medial malleolus, at the midline of the medial surface of the tibia.

Indications：urination disturbance, enuresis, hernia, irregular menstruation, morbid leukorrhea, pruritus vulvae, muscular atrophy or pain of the leg.

LR6 中都 ZhōngDū（郄穴）

位置　小腿内侧，内踝尖上 7 寸，胫骨内侧面的中央。

主治　腹痛，胁痛，泄泻，疝气，崩漏，恶露不绝。

Location：7 cun above the tip of the medial malleolus, at the midline of the medial surface of the tibia.

Indications: abdominal pain, hypochondriac pain, diarrhea, hernia, uterine bleeding, prolonged lochia.

LR7 膝关 XīGuān

位置　膝部,胫骨内侧髁的下方,阴陵泉(SP9)后 1 寸。

主治　膝部疼痛。

Location: inferior to the medial condyle of the tibia, 1 cun posterior to YinLíngQuán(SP9).

Indications: knee pain.

LR8 曲泉 QūQuán(合穴)

位置　膝部,腘横纹内侧端,半腱肌肌腱内缘凹陷中。

主治　小腹痛,小便不利,遗精,外阴疼痛,阴挺,阴痒,膝股内侧痛。

Location: at the medial end of the transverse crease of the popliteal fossa, in the depression at the medial border of the tendon of m. semitendinosus.

Indications: lower abdominal pain, urination disturbance, nocturnal emission, pain in the external genitalia prolapse of uterus, pruritus vulvae, pain in the medial aspect of the thigh and knee.

LR

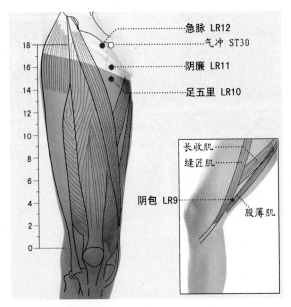

18 — 急脉 LR12
气冲 ST30
16 — 阴廉 LR11
14 — 足五里 LR10
12 —
10 —
8 —
6 —
长收肌
缝匠肌
4 — 阴包 LR9
股薄肌
2 —
0 —

LR9 阴包 YīnBāo

位置　股前区,髌骨上 4 寸,股薄肌与缝匠肌之间。

主治　腰骶引小腹痛,小便不利,遗尿,月经不调。

Location：at the medial aspect of the thigh, 4 cun above the patella, between the vastus medialis muscle and the sartorius muscle.

Indications：pain in the lumbosacral region referring to the lower abdomen, urination disturbance, enuresis, irregular menstruation.

LR10 足五里 ZúWǔLǐ

位置　股前区,气冲(ST30)直下 3 寸,动脉搏动处。

主治　小腹胀满,小便不通。

Location：in the anterior aspect of the thigh, 3 cun directly below QìChōng(ST30), where the pulsation of the artery is palpable.

Indications: lower abdominal distension and fullness, retention of urine.

LR11 阴廉 YīnLián
位置　股前区,气冲(ST30)直下 2 寸。
主治　月经不调,带下,小腹痛,腿股痛。

Location: in the anterior aspect of the thigh, 2 cun directly below QìChōng(ST30).

Indications: irregular menstruation, morbid leukorrhea, lower abdominal pain, pain in the thigh or leg.

LR12 急脉 JíMài
位置　腹股沟区,横平耻骨联合上缘,前正中线旁开 2.5 寸。
主治　少腹痛,阴部痛,疝气。

Location: in the inguinal groove, at the level of the upper border of symphysis pubis, 2.5 cun lateral to the anterior midline.

Indications: pain in the sides of the lower abdomen, pain in the external genitalia, hernia.

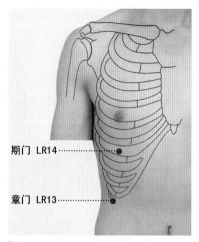

期门 LR14

章门 LR13

LR13 章门 ZhāngMén(脾募穴,脏会穴)

位置 侧腹部,当第 11 肋游离端的下际。

主治 胁痛,腹胀,肠鸣,呕吐,泄泻,完谷不化。

Location: in the lateral side of the abdomen, below the free end of the eleventh rib.

Indications: pain in the hypochondriac region, abdominal distension, borborygmus, vomiting, diarrhea, indigestion.

LR14 期门 QīMén(肝募穴)

位置 胸部,第 6 肋间隙,前正中线旁开 4 寸。

主治 胁痛,腹胀,呃逆,吐酸,乳痈,郁证,热病。

Location: in the sixth intercostal space, 4 cun lateral to the anterior midline.

Indications: pain in the hypochondriac region, abdominal distension, hiccup, acid regurgitation, mastitis, depression, febrile diseases.

13. 督脉 Governor Vessel

督脉分寸歌

督脉廿八行脊梁,尾闾骨端是长强。
二十一椎腰俞位,十六阳关细推详。
十四命门与脐对,十三悬枢在其乡。
十一椎下脊中穴,十椎之下中枢藏。
九椎之下筋缩取,七椎之下乃至阳。
六灵五神三身柱,陶道第一惟下方。
一椎之上大椎裕,入发五分哑门行。
风府一寸宛中取,脑户二五枕上量。
发上四寸强间位,五寸五分后顶强。
七寸百会顶上取,前行一尺囟会量。
一尺一寸上星会,入发五分神庭当。
鼻尖准头素髎穴,两眉中间穿印堂。
水沟鼻下人中正,兑端唇尖端上详。
龈交上齿龈缝处,齿龈连绵交互相。

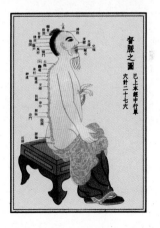

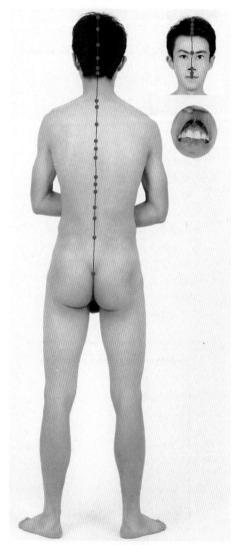

督脉

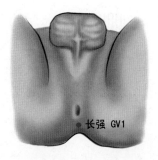

长强 GV1

GV1 长强 ChángQiáng(络穴)

位置 会阴区,尾骨下方,尾骨端与肛门连线的中点处。

主治 泄泻,便血,痔疾,脱肛,便秘,腰背痛,痫证。

Location：in the perineum, inferior to the coccyx, midway between the tip of coccyx and the anus.

Indications：diarrhea, hematochezia, hemorrhoids, prolapses of rectum, constipation, pain in the low back, epilepsy.

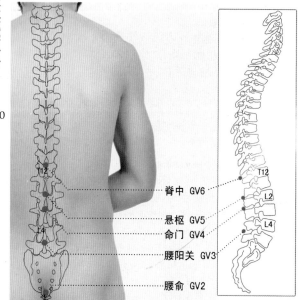

脊中 GV6

悬枢 GV5
命门 GV4

腰阳关 GV3

腰俞 GV2

GV2 腰俞 YāoShū

位置　骶区，正对骶管裂孔，后正中线上。

主治　月经不调，腰背强痛，痔疾，下肢痿痹，痫证。

Location：in the sacrum, at the hiatus of the sacrum, in the posterior midline

Indications：irregular menstruation, pain and stiffness of the low back, hemorrhoids, muscular atrophy or pain in the lower limbs, epilepsy.

GV3 腰阳关 YāoYángGuān

位置　脊柱区，第 4 腰椎棘突下凹陷中，后正中线上。

主治　月经不调，遗精，阳痿，腰骶痛，下肢痿痹。

Location：below the spinous process of the fourth lumbar vertebra, in the posterior midline.

Indications：irregular menstruation, nocturnal emission, impotence, pain in the lumbosacral region, muscular atrophy or pain in the lower limbs.

GV4 命门 MìngMén

位置 脊柱区,第 2 腰椎棘突下凹陷中,后正中线上。

主治 脊强,腰痛,阳痿,遗精,月经不调,带下,泄泻,带下。

Location:below the spinous process of the second lumbar vertebra,in the posterior midline.

Indications:stiffness of the back,lumbago,impotence,nocturnal emission,irregular menstruation,morbid leukorrhea,diarrhea,morbid leukorrhea.

GV5 悬枢 XuánShū

位置 脊柱区,第 1 腰椎棘突下凹陷中,后正中线上。

主治 腰背强痛,泄泻,完谷不化。

Location:below the spinous process of the first lumbar vertebra,in the posterior midline.

Indications:pain and stiffness of the back,diarrhea,indigestion.

GV6 脊中 JǐZhōng

位置 脊柱区,第 11 胸椎棘突下凹陷中,后正中线上。

主治 胃脘痛,腹泻,黄疸,痫证,腰背强痛。

Location:below the spinous process of the eleventh thoracic vertebra,in the posterior midline.

Indications:pain in the epigastric region,diarrhea,jaundice,epilepsy,stiffness and pain of the back.

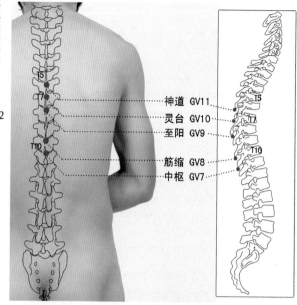

神道 GV11
灵台 GV10
至阳 GV9
筋缩 GV8
中枢 GV7

GV7 中枢 ZhōngShū

位置 脊柱区,第 10 胸椎棘突下凹陷中,后正中线上。

主治 胃脘痛,腰痛,脊强。

Location: below the spinous process of the tenth thoracic vertebra, in the posterior midline.

Indications: pain in the epigastric region, lumbago, stiffness of the back.

GV8 筋缩 JīnSuō

位置 脊柱区,第 9 胸椎棘突下凹陷中,后正中线上。

主治 痫证,脊强,胃痛。

Location: below the spinous process of the ninth thoracic vertebra, in the posterior midline.

Indications: epilepsy, stiffness of the back, gastric pain.

GV9 至阳 ZhìYáng

位置　脊柱区,第7胸椎棘突下凹陷中,后正中线上。

主治　黄疸,咳喘,脊强,胸背痛。

Location：below the spinous process of the seventh thoracic vertebra, in the posterior midline.

Indications：jaundice, cough, asthma, stiffness of the back, pain in the chest and back.

GV10 灵台 LíngTái

位置　脊柱区,第6胸椎棘突下凹陷中,后正中线上。

主治　咳嗽,气喘,疔疮,背痛项强。

Location：below the spinous process of the sixth thoracic vertebra, in the posterior midline.

Indications：cough, asthma, furuncles, back pain, neck rigidity.

GV11 神道 ShénDào

位置　脊柱区,第5胸椎棘突下凹陷中,后正中线上。

主治　健忘,惊悸,脊背强痛,咳嗽,心痛。

Location：below the spinous process of the fifth thoracic vertebra, in the posterior midline.

Indications：poor memory, palpitation, pain and stiffness of the back, cough, cardiac pain.

GV

大椎 GV14
陶道 GV13
身柱 GV12

GV12 身柱 ShēnZhù

位置 脊柱区,第3胸椎棘突下凹陷中,后正中线上。

主治 咳嗽,气喘,癫证,腰背强痛,疗疮。

Location: below the spinous process of the third thoracic vertebra, in the posterior midline.

Indications: cough, asthma, epilepsy, pain and stiffness of the back, furuncles.

GV13 陶道 TáoDào

位置 脊柱区,第1胸椎棘突下凹陷中,后正中线上。

主治 脊强,头痛,疟疾,热病。

Location: below the spinous process of the first thoracic vertebra, in the posterior midline.

Indications: stiffness of the back, headache, malaria, febrile diseases.

GV14 大椎 DàZhuī

位置 脊柱区,第 7 颈椎棘突下凹陷中,后正中线上。

主治 头项强痛,热病,骨蒸潮热,咳嗽,气喘,感冒,脊背强急。

Location: below the spinous process of the seventh cervical vertebra, in the posterior midline.

Indications: neck pain and rigidity, febrile diseases, afternoon fever, cough, asthma, common cold, stiffness of the back.

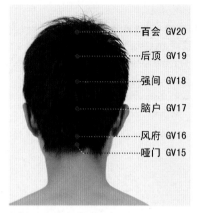

········百会 GV20

········后顶 GV19

········强间 GV18

········脑户 GV17

········风府 GV16

········哑门 GV15

GV15 哑门 YǎMén

位置 后颈区,第 2 颈椎棘突上际凹陷中,后正中线上。

主治 癫狂,痫证,聋哑,暴喑,中风,舌强不语,后头痛,项强。

Location: in the depression superior to the spinous process of the second cervical vertebra, in the posterior midline.

Indications: mental disorder, epilepsy, deafness and mute, sudden loss of voice, apoplexy, aphasia due to stiffness of the tongue, occipital headache, neck rigidity.

GV16 风府 FēngFǔ

位置 后颈区,枕外隆凸直下,两侧斜方肌之间凹陷中。

主治 头痛,项强,目眩,鼻衄,咽喉肿痛,中风不语、半身不遂,癫狂。

Location: directly below the external occipital protuberance, in the depression between m. trapezius of both sides.

Indications: headache, neck rigidity, blurred vision, epistaxis, sore throat, post-apoplexy aphasia, hemiplegia, mental disorder.

GV17 脑户 NǎoHù

位置 头部,枕外隆凸的上缘凹陷中。

主治 头晕,颈项强痛。

Location: in the depression at the upper border of the external occipital protuberance.

Indications: dizziness, pain and stiffness of the neck.

GV18 强间 QiángJiān

位置　头部,后发际正中直上 4 寸。

主治　头痛,项强,目眩,癫狂。

Location: 4 cun directly above the midpoint of the posterior hairline.

Indications: headache, neck rigidity, blurred vision, mental disorder.

GV19 后顶 HòuDǐng

位置　头部,后发际正中直上 5.5 寸。

主治　头痛,眩晕,癫狂,痫证。

Location: 5.5 cun directly above the midpoint of the posterior hairline.

Indications: headache, dizziness, vertigo, mental disorder, epilepsy.

GV20 百会 BǎiHuì

位置　头部,前发际正中直上 5 寸。

主治　头痛,眩晕,耳鸣,鼻塞,中风失语,昏厥,癫狂,脱肛,阴挺。

Location: 5 cun directly above the midpoint of the anterior hairline.

Indications: headache, dizziness, vertigo, tinnitus, nasal obstruction, aphasia by apoplexy, coma, mental disorder, prolapse of rectum or uterus.

神庭 GV24
上星 GV23
囟会 GV22
前顶 GV21
百会 GV20

GV21 前顶 QiánDǐng

位置 头部，前发际正中直上 3.5 寸。

主治 痫证，头晕，目眩，头顶痛，鼻渊。

Location：3.5 cun directly above the midpoint of the anterior hairline.

Indications：epilepsy, dizziness, vertigo, pain in the vertex, rhinorrhea.

GV22 囟会 XìnHuì

位置 头部，前发际正中直上 2 寸。

主治 头痛，目眩，鼻渊，小儿惊痫。

Location：2 cun above the midpoint of the anterior hairline.

Indications：headache, vertigo, rhinorrhea, infantile convulsion.

GV23 上星 ShàngXīng

位置 头部，前发际正中直上 1 寸。

主治 头痛，目痛，鼻衄，鼻渊，癫狂。

Location：1 cun directly above the midpoint of the anterior hairline.

Indications： headache, ophthalmalgia, epistaxis, rhinorrhea, mental disorder.

GV24 神庭 ShénTíng

位置 头部，前发际正中直上 0.5 寸。

主治 痫证，惊悸，失眠，头痛，眩晕，鼻渊。

Location：0.5 cun directly above the midpoint of the anterior hairline.

Indications： epilepsy, palpitation, insomnia, headache, dizziness, vertigo, rhinorrhea.

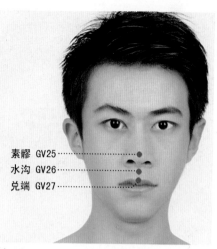

素髎 GV25
水沟 GV26
兑端 GV27

GV25 素髎 SùLiáo

位置 面部,鼻尖的正中央。

主治 昏厥,鼻塞,鼻衄,鼻渊,酒皶鼻。

Location:at the center in the tip of the nose.

Indications: loss of consciousness, nasal obstruction, epistaxis, rhinorrhea, rosacea.

GV26 水沟 ShuǐGōu

位置 面部,人中沟的上 1/3 与中 1/3 交点处。

主治 癫狂,痫证,小儿惊风,中风昏迷,昏厥,牙关紧闭,口眼歪斜,腰背强痛。

Location: at the junction of the upper one-third and middle two-thirds of the philtrum.

Indications: mental disorder, epilepsy, infantile convulsion, coma, trismus, facial paralysis, pain and stiffness of the low back.

GV27 兑端 DuìDuān

位置 面部,当上唇的尖端,人中沟下端的皮肤与唇的移行部。

主治 癫狂,齿龈肿痛。

Location: in the labial tubercle of the upper lip, at the vermilion border between the philtrum and upper lip.

Indications: mental disorder, swelling and pain of the gums.

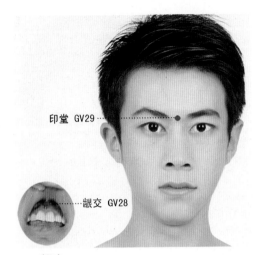

印堂 GV29

龈交 GV28

GV28 龈交 YínJiāo

位置 上唇内,上唇系带与上牙龈的交点。

主治 癫狂,齿龈肿痛,鼻渊。

Location：inside the upper lip, at the junction of the frenulum of the upper lip and the gum.

Indications：mental disorder, swelling and pain of the gums, rhinorrhea.

GV29 印堂 YìnTáng

位置 头部,两眉毛内侧端中间的凹陷中。

主治 头痛,头重,鼻衄,鼻渊,小儿惊风,前额疼痛,失眠。

Location：in the depression at the midway between the medial ends of the two eyebrows.

Indications：headache, heavy sensation of the head, epistaxis, rhinorrhea, infantile convulsion, pain in the forehead, insomnia.

14. 任脉 Conception Vessel

任脉分寸歌

任脉会阴两阴间，曲骨毛际陷中安。
中极脐下四寸取，关元脐下三寸连。
脐下二寸石门是，脐下寸半气海全。
脐下一寸阴交穴，脐之中央神阙观。
脐上一寸为水分，脐上二寸下脘连。
脐上三寸名建里，脐上四寸中脘焉。
脐上五寸上脘在，脐上六寸巨阙传。
鸠尾蔽骨下半寸，中庭膻下六铨。
膻中两乳之间是，膻上寸六玉堂联。
膻上紫宫三寸二，膻上四八华盖骈。
膻上璇玑六寸四，玑上一寸天突穿。
廉泉颔下结上已，承浆下唇中颐前。

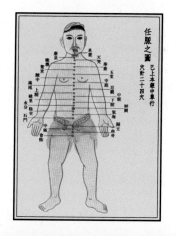

Chapter II Acupoints of 14 Meridians

第2章 十四经腧穴 ·

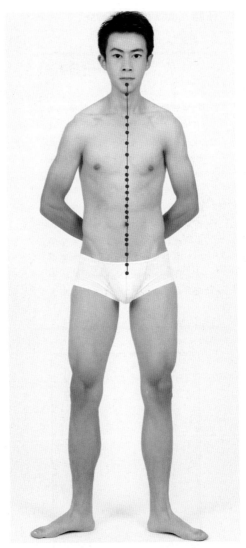

任脉

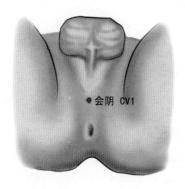

会阴 CV1

CV1 会阴 HuiYīn

位置 会阴区,男性在阴囊根部与肛门连线的中点,女性在大阴唇后联合与肛门连线的中点。

主治 阴痒,小便不利,痔疾,遗精,遗尿,月经不调,癫狂。

Location: between the anus and the root of the scrotum in males or between the anus and the posterior labia commissure in females.

Indications: pruritus vulvae, urination disturbance, enuresis, hemorrhoids, nocturnal emission, irregular menstruation, mental disorder.

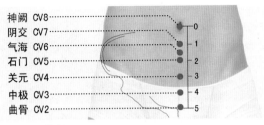

神阙 CV8 — 0
阴交 CV7 — 1
气海 CV6 — 2
石门 CV5 — 3
关元 CV4 — 4
中极 CV3
曲骨 CV2 — 5

CV2 曲骨 QūGǔ

位置 下腹部,耻骨联合上缘,前正中线上。

主治 小便不通,遗尿,遗精,阳痿,赤白带下,月经不调,痛经,疝气。

Location: at the midpoint of the upper border of the symphysis pubis, in the anterior midline.

Indications: retention of urine, enuresis, nocturnal emission, impotence, morbid leukorrhea, irregular menstruation, dysmenorrhea, hernia.

CV3 中极 ZhōngJí(膀胱募穴)

位置 下腹部,当脐中下4寸,前正中线上。

主治 遗尿,遗精,阳痿,崩漏,月经不调,小便频数,小腹痛,阴痒。

Location: in the lower abdomen, 4 cun below the umbilicus, in the anterior midline.

Indications: enuresis, nocturnal emission, impotence, uterine bleeding, irregular menstruation, frequency of urination, pain in the lower abdomen, pruritus vulvae.

CV

CV4 关元 GuānYuán(小肠募穴)

位置 下腹部,当脐中下3寸,前正中线上。

主治 遗精,遗尿,小便频数,月经不调,痛经,闭经,带下,崩漏,阴挺,疝气,小腹痛,脱肛,中风脱证。

Location: in the lower abdomen, 3 cun below the umbilicus, in the anterior midline.

Indications: nocturnal emission, enuresis, frequency of urination, irregular menstruation, dysmenorrhea, amenorrhea, morbid leukorrhea, uterine bleeding, prolapse of uterus, hernia, lower abdominal pain, prolapse of rectum, flaccid type of apoplexy.

CV5 石门 ShíMén(三焦募穴)

位置 下腹部,当脐中下 2 寸,前正中线上。

主治 腹痛,泄泻,水肿,疝气,尿闭,遗尿,闭经,带下,崩漏,产后出血。

Location:in the lower abdomen, 2 cun below the umbilicus, in the anterior midline.

Indications:abdominal pain, diarrhea, edema, hernia, retention of urine, enuresis, amenorrhea, morbid leukorrhea, uterine bleeding, postpartum hemorrhage.

CV6 气海 QìHǎi

位置 下腹部,当脐中下 1.5 寸,前正中线上。

主治 腹痛,遗精,疝气,水肿,痢疾,崩漏,月经不调,带下,产后出血,便秘,中风脱证,气喘。

Location:in the lower abdomen, 1.5 cun below the umbilicus, in the anterior midline.

Indications:abdominal pain, nocturnal emission, hernia, edema, dysentery, uterine bleeding, irregular menstruation, morbid leukorrhea, postpartum hemorrhage, constipation, flaccid type of apoplexy, asthma.

CV7 阴交 YīnJiāo

位置 下腹部,当脐中下 1 寸,前正中线上。

主治 腹胀,水肿,疝气,月经不调,崩漏,带下,产后出血,脐周痛。

Location:in the lower abdomen, 1 cun below the umbilicus, in the anterior midline.

Indications:abdominal distension, edema, hernia, irregular menstruation, uterine bleeding, morbid leukorrhea, postpartum hemorrhage, abdominal pain around the umbilicus.

CV8 神阙 ShénQuè

位置 脐区,脐中央。

主治 腹痛,肠鸣,中风脱证,脱肛,泄泻不止。

Location:in the centre of the umbilicus.

Indications:abdominal pain, borborygmus, flaccid type of apoplexy, prolapse of rectum, continuous diarrhea.

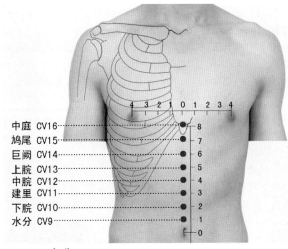

中庭 CV16
鸠尾 CV15
巨阙 CV14
上脘 CV13
中脘 CV12
建里 CV11
下脘 CV10
水分 CV9

CV9 水分 ShuǐFēn

位置 上腹部,脐中上1寸,前正中线上。

主治 腹痛,肠鸣,水肿,小便不通,泄泻。

Location: in the upper abdomen, 1 cun above the umbilicus, in the anterior midline.

Indications: abdominal pain, borborygmus, edema, retention of urine, diarrhea.

CV10 下脘 XiàWǎn

位置 上腹部,脐中上2寸,前正中线上。

主治 胃脘痛,腹痛,肠鸣,完谷不化,呕吐,泄泻。

Location: in the upper abdomen, 2 cun above the umbilicus, in the anterior midline.

Indications: epigastric pain, abdominal pain, borborygmus, indigestion, vomiting, diarrhea.

CV11 建里 JiànLǐ

位置 上腹部,脐中上3寸,前正中线上。

主治 胃痛,呕吐,腹胀,肠鸣,水肿,食欲不振。

Location: in the upper abdomen, 3 cun above the umbilicus, in the anterior midline.

Indications: gastric pain, vomiting, abdominal distension, borborygmus, edema, poor appetite.

CV

CV12 中脘 ZhōngWǎn(胃募穴、腑会穴)

位置　上腹部,脐中上 4 寸,前正中线上。

主治　胃痛,腹胀,肠鸣,反胃,吞酸,呕吐,泄泻,痢疾,黄疸,完谷不化,失眠。

Location: in the upper abdomen, 4 cun above the umbilicus, in the anterior midline.

Indications: gastric pain, abdominal distension, borborygmus, nausea, acid regurgitation, vomiting, diarrhea, dysentery, jaundice, indigestion, insomnia.

CV13 上脘 ShàngWǎn

位置　上腹部,脐中上 5 寸,前正中线上。

主治　胃痛,腹胀,反胃,呕吐,痫证,失眠。

Location: in the upper abdomen, 5 cun above the umbilicus, in the anterior midline.

Indications: gastric pain, abdominal distension, nausea, vomiting, epilepsy, insomnia.

CV14 巨阙 JùQuè(心募穴)

位置　上腹部,脐中上 6 寸,前正中线上。

主治　心胸痛,反胃,噎膈,泛酸,呕吐,癫狂,痫证,心悸。

Location: in the upper abdomen, 6 cun above the umbilicus, in the anterior midline.

Indications: pain in the cardiac region and the chest, nausea, dysphagia, acid regurgitation, vomiting, mental disorder, epilepsy, palpitation.

CV15 鸠尾 JiūWěi(络穴)

位置　上腹部,胸剑结合部下 1 寸,前正中线上。

主治　心胸痛,反胃,癫狂,痫证。

Location: in the upper abdomen, 1 cun below the xiphosternal synchondrosis, in the anterior midline.

Indications: pain in the cardiac region and the chest, nausea, mental disorder, epilepsy.

CV16 中庭 ZhōngTíng

位置　上腹部,胸剑结合中点处,前正中线上。

主治　胸胁胀满,噎膈,反胃,饮食不下。

Location: in the upper abdomen, midpoint of the xiphosternal synchondrosis, in the anterior midline.

Indications: distension and fullness in the chest and hypochondrium, dysphagia, nausea.

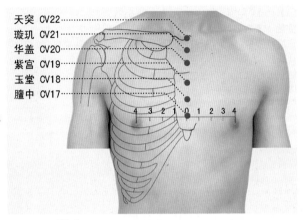

天突 CV22
璇玑 CV21
华盖 CV20
紫宫 CV19
玉堂 CV18
膻中 CV17

CV17 膻中 DànZhōng (心包募穴、气会穴)

位置 胸部,横平第 4 肋间隙,前正中线上。

主治 气喘,胸痛,胸闷,心悸,乳汁少,呃逆,噎膈。

Location: in the chest, at the level of the fourth intercostal space, in the anterior midline.

Indications: asthma, pain in the chest, oppressing feeling in the chest, palpitation, insufficient lactation, hiccup, dysphagia.

CV18 玉堂 YùTáng

位置 胸部,横平第 3 肋间隙,前正中线上。

主治 胸痛,咳嗽,气喘。

Location: in the chest, at the level of the third intercostal space, in the anterior midline.

Indications: pain in the chest, cough, asthma, vomiting.

CV19 紫宫 ZǐGōng

位置 胸部,横平第 2 肋间隙,前正中线上。

主治 胸痛,咳嗽,气喘。

Location: in the chest, at the level of the second intercostal space, in the anterior midline.

Indications: pain in the chest, cough, asthma.

CV

CV20 华盖 HuáGài

位置 胸部,横平第1肋间隙,前正中线上。

主治 胸胁胀痛,气喘,咳嗽。

Location: in the chest, at the level of the first intercostal space, in the anterior midline.

Indications: distending pain in the chest and hypochondrium, asthma, cough.

CV21 璇玑 XuánJī

位置 胸部,胸骨上窝下1寸,前正中线上。

主治 胸痛,咳嗽,气喘。

Location: in the chest, 1 cun below the suprasternal fossa, in the anterior midline.

Indications: pain in the chest, cough, asthma.

CV22 天突 TiānTū

位置 颈前区,胸骨上窝中央,前正中线上。

主治 哮喘,咳嗽,咽喉肿痛,咽干,呃逆,暴喑,瘿瘤,噎膈。

Location: in the anterior aspect of the neck, at the centre of the suprasternal fossa, in the anterior midline.

Indications: asthma, cough, sore throat, dry throat, hiccup, sudden loss of voice, goiter, dysphagia.

承浆 CV24

廉泉 CV23

CV23 廉泉 LiánQuán

位置 颈前区，喉结上方，舌骨上缘凹陷中，前正中线上。

主治 舌下肿痛，舌缓流涎，中风舌强不语，暴喑，吞咽困难。

Location：in the anterior aspect of the neck, superior to the prominentia laryngea, in the depression at the upper border of the hyoid bone, in the anterior midline.

Indications：swelling and pain of the subglossal region, hypersalivation with glossoplegia, aphasia with stiffness of tongue by apoplexy, sudden loss of voice, dysphagia.

CV24 承浆 ChéngJiāng

CV

位置 面部，颏唇沟的正中凹陷处。

主治 面肿，龈肿，齿痛，流涎，癫狂，口眼歪斜。

Location：in the face, in the depression at the centre of the mentolabial groove.

Indications：facial swelling, swelling of the gums, toothache, hypersalivation, mental disorder, facial paralysis.

第 3 章
Chapter III

经外奇穴
Extra Points

1. 头颈部穴 Head and Neck

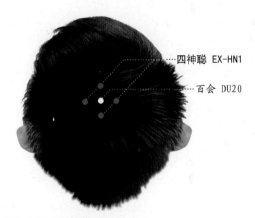

四神聪 EX-HN1

百会 DU20

EX-HN1 四神聪 SìShénCōng

位置 头部，百会(GV20)前后左右各旁开 1 寸，共 4 穴。

主治 头痛，眩晕，失眠，健忘，痫证。

Location：at the vertex, a group of 4 points, 1 cun respectively posterior, anterior and lateral to BǎiHuì(GV20).

Indications：headache, dizziness, vertigo, insomnia, poor memory, epilepsy.

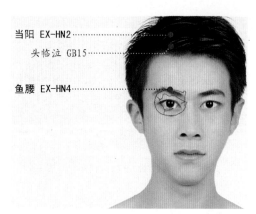

当阳 EX-HN2

头临泣 GB15

鱼腰 EX-HN4

EX – HN2 当阳 DāngYáng

位置 头前部,瞳孔直上,前发际上1寸。

主治 疏风通络,清头明目。

Location：in the forehead，directly above the pupil，1 cun within the anterior hairline.

Indications：to expel wind，promote circulation in collaterals or the head，improve acuity of vision.

EX – HN4 鱼腰 YúYāo

位置 头部,瞳孔直上,眉毛中。

主治 眉棱骨痛,眼睑瞤动,眼睑下垂,目翳,目赤肿痛。

Location：in the head，directly above the pupil，at the midpoint of the eyebrow.

Indications：pain in the supraorbital region，twitching or ptosis of the eyelids，cloudiness of the cornea，redness，swelling and pain of the eyes.

EX

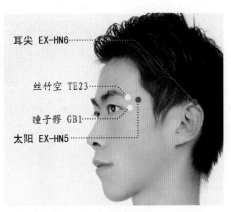

耳尖 EX-HN6

丝竹空 TE23

瞳子髎 GB1

太阳 EX-HN5

EX－HN5 太阳 TàiYáng

位置　头部,眉梢与目外眦之间,向后约一横指的凹陷中。

主治　头痛,目疾,口眼歪斜。

Location：in the head, in the depression about one Finger breadth posterior to the midpoint between the lateral end of the eyebrow and the outer canthus.

Indications：headache, eye diseases, facial paralysis.

EX－HN6 耳尖 ĚrJiān

位置　耳区,在外耳轮的最高点。

主治　目赤肿痛,热病,目翳。

Location：in the auricular area, at the apex of the helix.

Indications：redness, swelling and pain of the eyes, febrile disease, nebula.

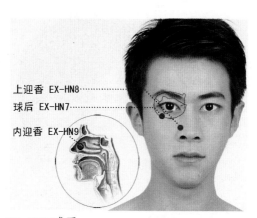

上迎香 EX-HN8
球后 EX-HN7
内迎香 EX-HN9

EX – HN7 球后 QiúHòu

位置　面部，眶下缘外 1/4 与内 3/4 交界处。

主治　目疾。

Location：in the face, at the junction of the lateral one-fourth and the medial three-fourths of the infraorbital margin.

Indications：eye diseases.

EX – HN8 上迎香 ShàngYíngXiāng

位置　面部，鼻翼软骨与鼻甲的交界处，近鼻翼沟上端处。

主治　鼻渊，鼻部疮疖。

Location：in the face, at the junction of the alar cartilage and the turbinate, in the upper end of alar groove.

Indications：rhinorrhea, skin ulcer or furuncle in the nose.

EX – HN9 内迎香 NèiYíngXiāng

位置　鼻孔内，鼻翼软骨与鼻甲交界的黏膜处。

主治　目赤肿，热病，中暑，鼻疾，喉痹，眩晕。

Location：inside the nostril, in the mucous membrane at the junction of the alar cartilage and the turbinate.

Indications：redness and swelling of eyes, febrile diseases, sunstroke, nasal diseases, pharyngitis, vertigo.

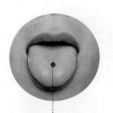
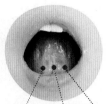

聚泉 EX-HN10

玉液 EX-HN13　金津 EX-HN12
海泉 EX-HN11

EX - HN10 聚泉 JùQuán

位置　口腔内,舌背正中缝的中点处。

主治　清散风热,祛邪开窍。

Location：in the oral cavity, midpoint of the median fissure in the dorsum of tongue.

Indications：to expel wind-heat, wake up the patient from unconsciousness.

EX - HN11 海泉 HǎiQuán

位置　口腔内,舌下系带中点处。

主治　祛邪开窍,生津止渴。

Location：in the oral cavity, midpoint of the frenulum of the tongue.

Indications：to wake up the patient from unconsciousness, promote the production of body fluid to quench thirst.

EX - HN12 金津 JīnJīn

位置　口腔内,舌下系带左侧的静脉上。

主治　舌肿,呕吐不止,舌强不语。

Location：in the oral cavity, on the left vein of the frenulum of the tongue.

Indications：swelling of the tongue, vomiting, aphasia with stiffness of tongue.

EX - HN13 玉液 YùYè

位置　口腔内,舌下系带右侧的静脉上。

主治　舌肿,呕吐不止,舌强不语。

Location：in the oral cavity, on the right vein of the frenulum of the tongue.

Indications：swelling of the tongue, vomiting, aphasia with stiffness of tongue.

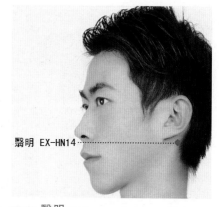

翳明 EX-HN14

EX - HN14 翳明 YìMíng

位置　颈部，翳风（TE17）后 1 寸。

主治　目疾，耳鸣，失眠。

Location：in the neck，1 cun posterior to YìFēng（TE17）．

Indications：eye diseases，tinnitus，insomnia．

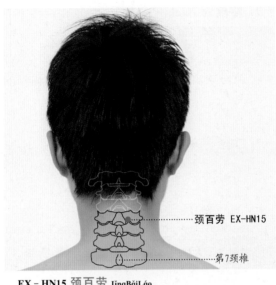

颈百劳 EX-HN15

第7颈椎

EX - HN15 颈百劳 JǐngBǎiLáo

位置　颈部,第7颈椎棘突直上2寸,后正中线旁开1寸。

主治　咳嗽,哮喘,落枕。

Location：in the neck, 2 cun above the spinous process of the seventh cervical vertebra, 1 cun lateral to the anterior midline.

Indications：cough, asthma, stiff neck.

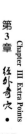

2. 背部穴 Back

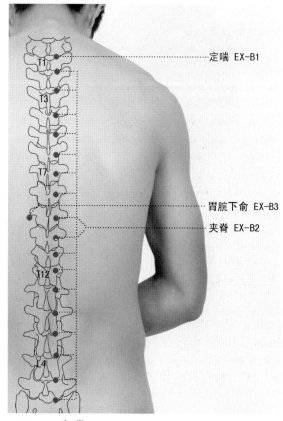

定喘 EX–B1

胃脘下俞 EX–B3

夹脊 EX–B2

EX - B1 定喘 DìngChuǎn

位置 脊柱区，横平第 7 颈椎棘突下，后正中线旁开 0.5 寸。

主治 哮喘，咳嗽，项强，肩背痛，风疹。

Location：in the vertebral column area，at the level of the lower border of the spinous process of the seventh cervical vertebra，0.5 cun lateral to the posterior midline.

Indications: asthma, cough, neck rigidity, pain in the shoulder and back, rubella.

EX - B2 夹脊 JiáJǐ

位置　脊柱区,第1胸椎至第5腰椎棘突下两侧,后正中线旁开0.5寸,一侧17穴。

主治　主调节脏腑机能。上背部穴位治疗心肺、上肢疾病;下背部穴位治疗胃肠疾病;腰部穴位治疗腰腹及下肢疾病。

Location: in the vertebral column area, at the level of the lower border of each spinous process from the first thoracic vertebra to the fifth lumbar vertebra, 0.5 cun lateral to the posterior midline, 17 on each side.

Indications: to regulate the Zangfu organs. Points in the upper chest treat diseases of the heart, lung or upper limbs. Points in the lower chest treat gastrointestinal diseases. Points in the lumbar treat diseases of the lumbar, abdomen or lower limbs.

EX - B3 胃脘下俞 WèiWǎnXiàShū

位置　脊柱区,横平第8胸椎棘突下,后正中线旁开1.5寸。

主治　消渴,呕吐,腹痛,胸胁痛。

Location: in the vertebral column area, at the level of he lower border of the spinous process of the eighth thoracic vertebra, 1.5 cun lateral to the posterior midline.

Indications: diabetes, vomiting, abdominal pain, pain in the chest and hypochondriac region.

EX

第3章　Chapter III Extra Points　经外奇穴　•

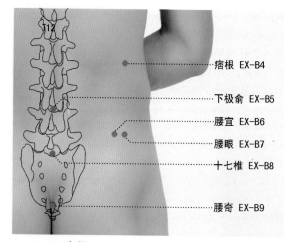

痞根 EX-B4

下极俞 EX-B5

腰宜 EX-B6

腰眼 EX-B7

十七椎 EX-B8

腰奇 EX-B9

EX‑B4 痞根 PǐGēn

位置 腰区,横平第1腰椎棘突下,后正中线旁开3.5寸。

主治 腹中痞块,腰痛。

Location：in the lumbar region, at the level of the lower border of the spinous process of the first lumbar vertebra, 3.5 cun lateral to the posterior midline.

Indications：mass in the abdomen, lumbar pain.

EX‑B5 下极俞 XiàJíShū

位置 腰区,第3腰椎棘突下。

主治 强腰健肾。

Location：in the lumbar region, below the spinous process of the third lumbar vertebra.

Indications：to strengthen the lumbar and the kidney.

EX‑B6 腰宜 YāoYí

位置 腰区,横平第4腰椎棘突下,后正中线旁开3寸。

主治 腰痛,月经不调。

Location：in the lumbar region, at the level of the lower border of the spinous process of the fourth lumbar vertebra, 3 cun lat-

EX

eral to the posterior midline.

Indications：lumbar pain，irregular menstruation.

EX－B7 腰眼 YāoYǎn

位置　腰区，横平第4腰椎棘突下，后正中线旁开约3.5寸凹陷中。

主治　腰痛，尿频，月经不调。

Location：in the lumbar region，at the level of the lower border of the spinous process of the fourth lumbar vertebra，in the depression about 3.5 cun lateral to the posterior midline.

Indications：lumbar pain，frequency of urination，irregular menstruation.

EX－B8 十七椎 ShíQīZhuī

位置　腰区，第5腰椎棘突下凹陷中。

主治　腰痛，腿痛，下肢痿痹，月经不调，痛经。

Location：in the lumbar region，in the depression below the spinous process of the fifth lumbar vertebra.

Indications：lumbar pain，pain in the lower limbs，paralysis of the lower limbs，irregular menstruation，dysmenorrhea.

EX－B9 腰奇 YāoQí

位置　骶区，尾骨端直上2寸，骶角之间凹陷中。

主治　痫证，头痛，失眠，便秘。

Location：in the sacrum，2 cun directly above the tip of the coccyx，in the depression between the sacral cornua.

Indications：epilepsy，headache，insomnia，constipation.

3. 胸腹部穴 Chest and Abdomen

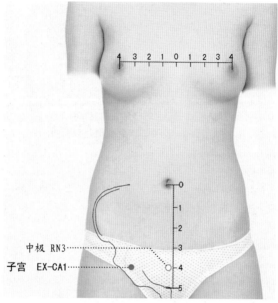

中极 RN3

子宫 EX-CA1

EX-CA1 子宫 ZiGōng

位置 下腹部,脐中下 4 寸,前正中线旁开 3 寸。

主治 阴挺,月经不调。

Location: in the lower abdomen, 4 cun below the umbilicus, 3 cun lateral to the anterior midline.

Indications: prolapse of uterus, irregular menstruation.

4. 上肢部穴 Upper Extremities

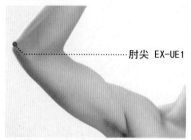

肘尖 EX-UE1

EX－UE1 肘尖 ZhǒuJiān

位置 肘后区,尺骨鹰嘴的尖端。

主治 瘰疬。

Location: in the posterior aspect of the elbow, at the tip of the olecranon of ulna.

Indications: scrofula.

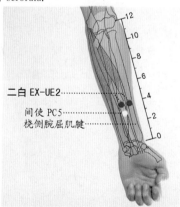

二白 EX-UE2

间使 PC5

桡侧腕屈肌腱

EX－UE2 二白 ÈrBái

位置 前臂前区,腕掌侧远端横纹上 4 寸,桡侧腕屈肌腱的两侧,一肢 2 穴。

主治 痔疮疼痛,脱肛。

Location: in the metacarpal aspect of the forearm, 4 cun above the transverse wrist crease, at the both sides of the tendon of m. flexor carpi radialis, two points on one forearm.

Indications: hemorrhoids, prolapse of rectum.

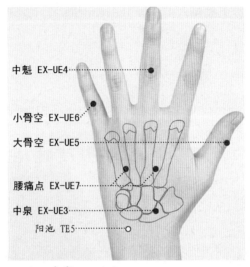

中魁 EX-UE4

小骨空 EX-UE6

大骨空 EX-UE5

腰痛点 EX-UE7

中泉 EX-UE3

阳池 TE5

EX – UE3 中泉 ZhōngQuán

位置　前臂后区,腕背侧远端横纹上,指总伸肌腱桡侧的凹陷中。

主治　胸闷,胃痛,吐血。

Location：in the dorsal aspect of the forearm, at the dorsal crease of the wrist, in the depression on the radial side of the tendon of common extensor muscle of Fingers.

Indications：oppressing feeling in the chest, gastric pain, hematemesis.

EX – UE4 中魁 ZhōngKuí

位置　中指,中指背面,近侧指间关节的中点处。

主治　反胃,呕吐,呃逆。

Location：at the midpoint of the proximal interphalangeal joint of the middle Finger at dorsum aspect.

Indications：nausea, vomiting, hiccup.

EX – UE5 大骨空 DàGǔKōng

位置　手指,拇指背面,指间关节的中点处。

主治　退翳明目。

Location：at the midpoint of the interphalangeal joint of the thumb at dorsum aspect.

Indications：to remove nebula, improve acuity of vision.

EX – UE6 小骨空 XiǎoGǔKōng

位置　手指,小指背面,近侧指间关节的中点处。

主治　明目止痛。

Location：at the midpoint of the proximal interphalangeal joint of the little finger at the dorsum aspect.

Indications：improve acuity of vision, relieve pain.

EX – UE7 腰痛点 YāoTòngDiǎn

位置　手背,第2、3掌骨及第4、5掌骨间,腕背侧远端横纹与掌指关节的中点处,一手2穴。

主治　腰扭伤。

Location：in the dorsum of hands, between the second and third metacarpal bones, and between the fourth and fifth metacarpal bones, midway between the transverse wrist crease and meta-carpophalangeal joint, two points in each hand.

Indications：acute lumbar sprain.

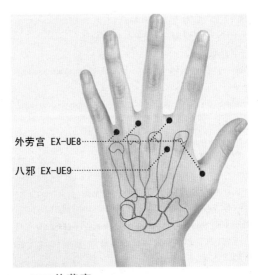

外劳宫 EX-UE8

八邪 EX-UE9

EX-UE8 外劳宫 WàiLáoGōng

位置 手背,第 2、3 掌骨间,掌指关节后 0.5 寸(指寸)凹陷中。

主治 通经活络,祛风止痛。

Location：in the dorsum of hand，between the second and third metacarpal bones，in the depression 0.5 cun distal to the metacarpophalangeal joint.

Indications：to promote circulation in the meridians and collaterals，expel wind，relieve pain.

EX-UE9 八邪 BāXié

位置 手背,第 1~5 指间,指蹼缘后方赤白肉际处,左右共 8 穴。

主治 烦热,手指麻木,手指拘挛,手背红肿。

Location：in the dorsum of hand，at the junction of the red and white skin distal to the web margins between the five Fingers，eight in all.

Indications：excessive heat，numbness of Fingers，spasm and spasm of the fingers，redness and swelling of the dorsum of hand.

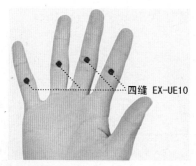

四缝 EX-UE10

EX - UE10 四缝 Sìfèng

位置 手指,第 2～5 指掌面的近侧指关节横纹的中央,一手 4 穴。

主治 小儿疳积,顿咳。

Location: in the fingers, at the midpoint of the transverse creases of the proximal interphalangeal joints of the index, middle, ring and little fingers, 4 points in each hand.

Indications: malnutrition and indigestion syndrome in children, whooping cough.

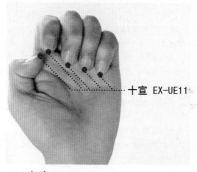

十宣 EX-UE11

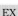

EX - UE11 十宣 Shíxuān

位置 手指,十指尖端,距指甲游离缘 0.1 寸(指寸),左右共 10 穴。

主治 中风,昏迷,痫证,高热,乳蛾,小儿惊风,指端麻木。

Location: at the tips of the ten fingers, about 0.1 cun distal to the nails, 10 points in both hands.

Indications: apoplexy, coma, epilepsy, high fever, acute tonsillitis, infantile convulsion, numbness of the finger tips.

5．下肢部穴 Lower Extremities

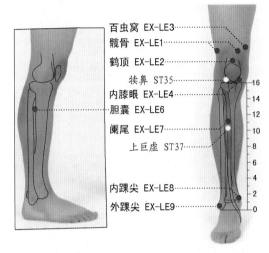

百虫窝 EX-LE3
髋骨 EX-LE1
鹤顶 EX-LE2
犊鼻 ST35
内膝眼 EX-LE4
胆囊 EX-LE6
阑尾 EX-LE7
上巨虚 ST37
内踝尖 EX-LE8
外踝尖 EX-LE9

EX – LE1 髋骨 KuānGǔ

位置　股前区，梁丘(ST34)两旁各 1.5 寸，一肢 2 穴。

主治　膝关节痛，中风偏瘫，腿疼痛无力，膝部红肿。

Location：in the anterior aspect of the thigh, 1.5 cun median and lateral to LiángQiū (ST34), 2 points in each thigh.

Indications：knee pain, hemiplegia, pain and weakness of the lower limbs, redness and swelling of the knee.

EX – LE2 鹤顶 HèDǐng

位置　膝前区，髌底中点的上方凹陷中。

主治　膝痛，足胫无力，瘫痪。

Location：in the anterior aspect of the knee, in the depression at the midpoint of the superior patellar border.

Indications：knee pain, weakness or paralysis of the leg and foot.

EX – LE3 百虫窝 BǎiChóngWō

位置　股前区，髌底内侧端上 3 寸。

主治　风疹，湿疹，虫积。

Location：in the anterior aspect of the knee, 3 cun above the mediosuperior border of the patella.

Indications：rubella, eczema, gastrointestinal parasitic diseases.

EX

EX - LE4 内膝眼 NèiXīYǎn

位置　膝部，髌韧带内侧凹陷处的中央。

主治　膝痛，下肢无力。

Location：in the knee, in the depression lateral to the patellar ligament.

Indications：knee pain, weakness of the lower limbs.

EX - LE6 胆囊 DǎnNáng

位置　小腿外侧，腓骨小头直下 2 寸。

主治　急、慢性胆囊炎、胆石症、胆道蛔虫症、下肢痿痹。

Location：in the lateral aspect of the leg, 2 cun directly below the head of fibula.

Indications：acute or chronic cholecystitis, cholelithiasis, biliary ascariasis, muscular atrophy or numbness of the lower limbs.

EX - LE7 阑尾 LánWěi

位置　小腿外侧，髌韧带外侧凹陷下 5 寸，胫骨前嵴外一横指（中指）。

主治　急、慢性阑尾炎，消化不良，下肢瘫痪。

Location：in the lateral aspect of the leg, 5 cun below the depression lateral to the patella ligament, one finger breath (middle finger) from the anterior border of the tibia.

Indications：acute or chronic appendicitis, indigestion, paralysis of the lower limbs.

EX - LE8 内踝尖 NèiHuáiJiān

位置　踝区，内踝的最凸起处。

主治　牙痛，小儿不语，转筋。

Location：at the tip of the medial malleolus.

Indications：toothache, children without a word, tendon transfer.

EX - LE9 外踝尖 WàiHuáiJiān

位置　踝区，外踝的最凸起处。

主治　脚趾拘急，踝关节肿痛，脚气，牙痛。

Location：at the tip of the external malleolus.

Indications：pain in the toes, swelling and pain in the dorsum of foot, beriberi, toothache.

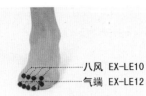

八风 EX-LE10
气端 EX-LE12

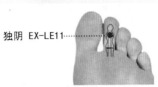

独阴 EX-LE11

EX - LE10 八风 **BāFēng**

位置 足背,第1~5趾间,趾蹼缘后方赤白肉际处,左右共8穴。

主治 脚气,趾痛,足背肿痛。

Location: in the dorsum of hand, at the junction of the red and white skin distal to the web margins between the five toes, eight in all.

Indications: beriberi, pain in the toes, swelling and pain in the dorsum of foot.

EX - LE11 独阴 **DúYīn**

位置 足底,第2趾的跖侧远侧趾间关节的中点。

主治 月经不调,胃痛,呕吐,心绞痛。

Location: in the sole, at the midpoint of the distal interphalangeal joint of the second toe.

Indications: irregular menstruation, gastric pain, vomiting, angina pectoris.

EX - LE12 气端 **QìDuān**

位置 足趾,十趾端的中央,距趾甲游离缘0.1寸(指寸),左右共10穴。

主治 脚气,足趾麻痹,足背红肿,急救。

Location: in the tips of the ten toes, about 0.1 cun distal to the nails, 10 points in both feet.

Indications: beriberi, toe paralysis, dorsal swelling, first aid.

EX

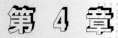

Chapter IV

耳穴
Auricular Points

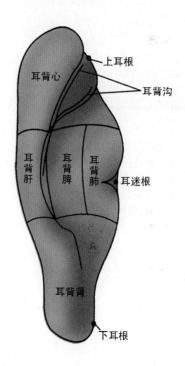

上耳根

耳背心

耳背沟

耳背肝

耳背脾

耳背肺

耳迷根

耳背肾

下耳根

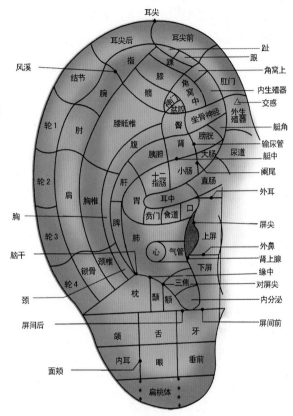

附录一 十四经腧穴名称索引

Appendix I Index of Acupoints of 14 Meridians

—— Z ——

附录二　经外奇穴名称索引
Appendix II　Index of Extra Points

附录三　腧穴部位速查

Appendix III　Index of Acupoints in Same Regions

一、头颈部 Head and Neck

1. 正面 Anterior Aspect

承泣 ST1	四白 ST2	巨髎 ST3	地仓 ST4	大迎 ST5
颊车 ST6	下关 ST7	头维 ST8	人迎 ST9	水突 ST10
气舍 ST11	缺盆 ST12	睛明 BL1	攒竹 BL2	眉冲 BL3
曲差 BL4	五处 BL5	瞳子髎 GB1	本神 GB13	阳白 GB14
头临泣 GB15	目窗 GB16	丝竹空 TE23	巨骨 LI16	天鼎 LI17
扶突 LI18	口禾髎 LI19	迎香 LI20	囟会 GV22	上星 GV23
神庭 GV24	素髎 GV25	水沟 GV26	兑端 GV27	印堂 GV29
天突 CV22	廉泉 CV23	承浆 CV24		

2. 背面 Posterior Aspect

百会 GV20	后顶 GV19	强间 GV18	脑户 GV17	风府 GV16
哑门 GV15	大椎 GV14	络却 BL8	玉枕 BL9	脑空 GB19
风池 GB20	天柱 BL10			

3. 头顶 Vertex

百会 GV20	前顶 GV21	囟会 GV22	上星 GV23	神庭 GV24
络却 BL8	通天 BL7	承灵 GB18	承光 BL6	正营 GB17
目窗 GB16	五处 BL5	头维 ST8	曲差 BL4	本神 GB13
头临泣 GB15	眉冲 BL3			

4. 侧面 Temple

正营 GB17	前顶 GV21	通天 BL7	百会 GV20	承灵 GB18
络却 BL8	后顶 GV19	强间 GV18	率谷 GB8	天冲 GB9
角孙 TE20	脑空 GB19	玉枕 BL9	脑户 GV17	浮白 GB10
颅息 TE19	头窍阴 GB11	风池 GB20	风府 GV16	天柱 BL10
哑门 GV15	瘈脉 TE18	完骨 GB12	天牖 TE16	天容 SI17
天窗 SI16	承光 BL6	囟会 GV22	目窗 GB16	五处 BL5
头临泣 GB15	上星 GV23	曲差 BL4	眉冲 BL3	神庭 GV24
本神 GB13	头维 ST8	颔厌 GB4	悬颅 GB5	阳白 GB14
悬厘 GB6	曲鬓 GB7	丝竹空 TE23	耳和髎 TE22	耳门 TE21
瞳子髎 GB1	上关 GB3	听宫 SI19	下关 ST7	听会 GB2
颧髎 SI18	口禾髎 LI19	翳风 TE17	颊车 ST6	大迎 ST5
浮突 LI18	人迎 ST9	天鼎 LI17	水突 ST10	

二、胸腹部经穴 Chest and Abdomen

1. 正面 Anterior Aspect

缺盆 ST12	气户 ST13	云门 LU2	中府 LU1	库房 ST14
周荣 SP20	屋翳 ST15	胸乡 SP19	膺窗 ST16	天溪 SP18
天池 PC1	乳中 ST17	食窦 SP17	乳根 ST18	期门 LR14
不容 ST19	承满 ST20	日月 GB24	梁门 ST21	关门 ST22
腹哀 SP16	太乙 ST23	滑肉门 ST24	天枢 ST25	大横 SP15
外陵 ST26	腹结 SP14	大巨 ST27	水道 ST28	五枢 GB27
维道 GB28	归来 ST29	府舍 SP13	冲门 SP12	急脉 LR12
气冲 ST30	俞府 KI27	彧中 KI26	天突 CV22	璇玑 CV21
华盖 CV20	神藏 KI25	紫宫 CV19	灵墟 KI24	玉堂 CV18
神封 KI23	膻中 CV17	步廊 KI22	中庭 CV16	鸠尾 CV15
幽门 KI21	巨阙 CV14	腹通谷 KI20	上脘 CV13	阴都 KI19
中脘 CV12	石关 KI18	建里 CV11	商曲 KI17	下脘 CV10
水分 CV9	肓俞 KI16	神阙 CV8	中注 KI15	阴交 CV7
气海 CV6	四满 KI14	石门 CV5	气穴 KI13	关元 CV4
大赫 KI12	中极 CV3	横骨 KI11	曲骨 CV2	

2. 侧胸腹部 Lateral Aspect

渊腋 GB22	辄筋 GB23	大包 SP21	日月 GB24	章门 LR13
京门 GB25	带脉 GB26	五枢 GB27	维道 GB28	

3. 背部 Back

肩中俞 SI15	肩外俞 SI14	肩井 GB21	附分 BL41	天髎 TE15
曲垣 SI13	肩髎 TE14	臑俞 SI10	秉风 SI12	魄户 BL42
膏肓 BL43	肩贞 SI9	天宗 SI11	神堂 BL44	谚语 BL45
膈关 BL46	魂门 BL47	阳纲 BL48	意舍 BL49	胃仓 BL50
肓门 BL51	志室 BL52	关元俞 BL26	小肠俞 BL27	膀胱俞 BL28
胞肓 BL53	中膂俞 BL29	秩边 BL54	白环俞 BL30	会阳 BL35
大椎 GV14	大杼 BL11	陶道 GV13	风门 BL12	肺俞 BL13
身柱 GV12	厥阴俞 BL14	心俞 BL15	神道 GV11	督俞 BL16
灵台 GV10	膈俞 BL17	至阳 GV9	肝俞 BL18	筋缩 GV8
胆俞 BL19	中枢 GV7	脾俞 BL20	脊中 GV6	胃俞 BL21
三焦俞 BL22	悬枢 GV5	肾俞 BL23	命门 GV4	气海俞 BL24
大肠俞 BL25	腰阳关 GV3	上髎 BL31	次髎 BL32	中髎 BL33
下髎 BL34	腰俞 GV2			

三、上肢部 Upper Extremities

1. 屈面(掌心所在一面)Flexing Aspect (Palmar Aspect)

天府 LU3	侠白 LU4	尺泽 LU5	孔最 LU6	列缺 LU7
经渠 LU8	太渊 LU9	鱼际 LU10	天泉 PC2	青灵 HT2
曲泽 PC3	少海 HT3	郄门 PC4	间使 PC5	内关 PC6
灵道 HT4	通里 HT5	阴郄 HT6	神门 HT7	大陵 PC7
劳宫 PC8	少府 HT8	中冲 PC9		

2. 外侧面 Lateral Aspect

肩髃 LI15	臂臑 LI14	手五里 LI13	肘髎 LI12	曲池 LI11
手三里 LI10	上廉 LI9	下廉 LI8	温溜 LI7	偏历 LI6
阳溪 LI5	合谷 LI4	三间 LI3	二间 LI2	

3. 伸面（手背所在一面）Extending Aspect（Dorsal Aspect）

肩髎 TE14	肩贞 SI9	臑会 TE13	消泺 TE12	清泠渊 TE11
天井 TE10	小海 SI8	四渎 TE9	支正 SI7	三阳络 TE8
会宗 TE7	支沟 TE6	外关 TE5	养老 SI6	阳池 TE4
阳谷 SI5	腕骨 SI4	中渚 TE3	液门 TE2	前谷 SI2

4. 井穴（位于手指、足趾，经气所出的输穴）Jing-Well Points, at the terminal phalanx of the fingers, where the meridian qi starts to bubble

关冲 TE1	少冲 HT9	少泽 SI1	商阳 LI1	中冲 PC9
少商 LU11				

四、下肢部 Lower Extremities

1. 前面 Anterior Aspect

髀关 ST31	伏兔 ST32	阴市 ST33	梁丘 ST34	犊鼻 ST35
足三里 ST36	上巨虚 ST37	条口 ST38	丰隆 ST40	下巨虚 ST39
解溪 ST41				

2. 内侧面 Medial Aspect

冲门 SP12	急脉 LR12	阴廉 LR11	足五里 LR10	箕门 SP1
阴包 LR9	血海 SP10	曲泉 LR8	阴陵泉 SP9	地机 SP8
中都 LR6	漏谷 SP7	蠡沟 LR5	三阴交 SP6	阴谷 KI10
膝关 LR7	筑宾 KI9	交信 KI8	复溜 KI7	

3. 背面 Posterior Aspect

承扶 BL36	殷门 BL37	浮郄 BL38	委阳 BL39	委中 BL40
合阳 BL55	承筋 BL56	承山 BL57	飞扬 BL58	跗阳 BL59
昆仑 BL60	阴谷 KI10			

4. 外侧面 Lateral Aspect

居髎 GB29	环跳 GB30	风市 GB31	中渎 GB32	膝阳关 GB2
阳陵泉 GB3	阳交 GB35	外丘 GB36	光明 GB37	阳辅 GB38
悬钟 GB39	丘墟 GB40			

5. 足背 Dorsum of Foot

丘墟 GB40	足临泣 GB41	地五会 GB42	侠溪 GB43	足窍阴 GB44
中封 LR4	解溪 ST41	冲阳 ST42	太冲 LR3	陷谷 ST43
行间 LR2	内庭 ST44	大敦 LR1	厉兑 ST45	

6. 足内侧 Medial Aspect of Foot

| 太溪 KI3 | 照海 KI6 | 大钟 KI4 | 水泉 KI5 | 然谷 KI2 |
| 隐白 SP1 | 大都 SP2 | 太白 SP3 | 公孙 SP4 | 商丘 SP5 |

7. 足外侧 Lateral Aspect of Foot

| 昆仑 BL60 | 申脉 BL62 | 仆参 BL61 | 金门 BL63 | 京骨 BL64 |
| 束骨 BL65 | 足通谷 BL66 | 至阴 BL67 | | |

8. 井穴(位于手指、足趾末端,经气所出的输穴) Jing-Well Points, at the terminal phalanx of the toes, where the meridian qi starts to bubble

| 至阴 BL67 | 足窍阴 GB44 | 大敦 LR1 | 隐白 SP1 | 厉兑 ST45 |
| 涌泉 KI1 | | | | |